MIND
OVER
MUSCLE

The Effortless Way to a Perfect Body

JAMES VILLEPIGUE, ACE

Coauthor of the bestselling *Body Sculpting Bible* series

HatherleighPress
New York   London

HatherleighPress
5-22 46th Avenue, Suite 200
Long Island City, NY 11101
www.hatherleighpress.com

Library of Congress Cataloging-in-Publication Data
Villepigue, James C.
    Mind over muscle : using the power of your mind to manifest the body of
your dreams / James Villepigue ; photographs by Peter Field Peck.
        p. cm.
Includes bibliographical references and index.
ISBN: 978-1-57826-223-6 (alk. paper)
    1. Bodybuilding--Psychological aspects. 2. Physical
    fitness—Psychological aspects. I. Title.
GV546.5.V548 2006
613.7'1019--dc22

                                        2006003635

ISBN 978-1-57826-223-6

Mind Over Muscle is available for bulk purchase, special promotions, and premiums. For information on reselling and special purchase opportunities, call 1-800-528-2550 and ask for the Special Sales Manager.

Special thanks to Steve Weinberger from Powerhouse Gym, 235-c Robbins Lane, Syosset, New York, 516-933-1111, www.bevfrancis.com

Interior design by Christine Weathersbee
Cover design by Deborah Miller

10 9 8 7 6 5 4 3 2 1
Printed in Canada

Acknowledgements

The *Mind Over Muscle* project is, without question, the most important and intense work I have ever accomplished. I would like to dedicate this most exciting project to the most important people in my life:

To my extraordinary mom, Nancy, I am truly blessed by God to be your son and I thank you for always being there to support me and never allow me to quit—I am truly amazed and inspired by your strength.

To my awesome sister, Deborah, these have been very difficult times for you, me, and mom. Our love and connection is what strength is defined by. As always, "So very proud of you!"

To my best pal and navigator through life, my dad, Jim, I love, adore, and honor you every moment of my life. I miss you so much, pal. God bless you!

To God, I am grateful to you for the strength, love and support you have blessed me with. Thank you, thank you, thank you.

To Heather, my beautiful wife, thank you for your incredible support and companionship. I love you, baby.

To all of my amazing family and friends: To Jason Giannetti, my best man and my best bro—I love you little brother! To Carl "Malone," your unconditional kindness is so appreciated and cannot be put into words—thank you for being such a great friend, bro! To Bobby Rusie, since we were young you have always been there to keep me laughing—thanks, my bro!

To my amazing grandparents, Gloria and Charlie, you are both such remarkably caring humanitarians and I love you. To my Aunt Joyce, Uncle Tony, and Cousin Joey, I love you and thank you for your incredible love and support. We needed you and you were right there!

To Hugo Rivera, my amazing bro and business partner, we have had a real journey so far and I look forward to our exciting future travels together. Thank you for your great support, your uplifting enthusiasm, and your friendship.

To Christopher Oliver, for his wonderful production work on the *Mind Over Muscle* audio CD.

To Steve Weinberger from Powerhouse Gym, where the photos were taken.

To our models, Anthony Cotilleta, Candice Holdorf, and Isobella Jade.

And a very special thanks to Lisa Trivell for contributing her expertise on the yoga section.

Additionally, I would like to thank the following people: My publishers and great friends, Andrew Flach and Kevin Moran: A heartfelt thanks for all of the wonderful opportunities we have shared and continue to share together. To my bro, Peter Field Peck, as always, amazing work—you are always the best part of the shoot! Alyssa, thank you for your hard work. Andrea, thank you so very much for your amazing support and incredible talent. Deborah, thank you—you are so awesome! To all of the Hatherleigh publishing team, you are all the very best—I look forward to great things to come.

Finally, to all of my incredible clients and readers, thank you so very much for your interest and support. These last couple of years have been the most difficult, yet most empowering, years of my life. Beyond measure, I appreciate you all! Please enjoy…Good luck and God Bless!

Instantly Download Your Free Custom Workout

Visit: www.mindovermusclebonus.com

When you get to the site, simply enter your name and e-mail address. I will immediately send you a questionnaire to create a fully customized workout plan that you can use in conjunction with the "Mind Over Muscle" program. I'll also give you a FREE subscription to my world-famous, no B.S., no hype *Mind Over Muscle* e-zine, plus a 40-page FREE report, *Unleashing Your Mind/Muscle Connection*! All these gifts are YOURS FREE as a thank you for purchasing my book.

I will only be offering this for a limited time, so please visit www.mindovermusclebonus.com right now.

Table of Contents

Foreword

When it comes to physical fitness, we tend to decompartmentalize our bodies from our minds. Exercise works the body, or so prevailing sentiment goes, "health" really means our physical well-being, and even eating properly has more to do with the stomach than it does the brain.

But healthy people have a secret, and they do not mind sharing it with you. Once you discover their secret, you will finally be able to achieve the toned and strong body, boundless energy, and glowing good health you've always craved. Their secret is not based on half-truths, emotions, or fads, but in fact has been the subject of medical research for many years, and the evidence confirms what those healthy people have known all along: Our thoughts, emotions, and attitude-in other words, our minds-play an important part in our physical health and well-being.

As the publisher of *MuscleMag International* and *Oxygen Women's Fitness* and as a participant in my youth in weightlifting and bodybuilding contests, I've seen it proven time and again. The best workout program in the world will do you no good until you put your mind into it. *Mind Over Muscle* will show you, step-by-step, exactly how to do that. Not only will you be amazed at the results, but you will have more fun with an exercise program than you ever have before. No matter what your fitness level, I highly recommend this book to help you reach physical perfection effortlessly.

—Robert Kennedy
Publisher, *MuscleMag International* and *Oxygen Women's Fitness*

Introduction:
Why Your Mind Matters

Let's face it: thousands of exercise and diet programs are available to the average consumer, and all of them seem to offer a different perspective on the best methods for losing weight and creating a perfect physique. To list them all here would be to date the book: from the Peanut Butter Diet to the Hollywood Star Diet, the names come and go so often that they might as well be a revolving door into which you throw your hard-earned money and hope for the best.

Regardless of where you're coming from, couch potato or fitness buff, gym rat or gym-a-phobic, you're obviously not satisfied with any of these programs or you wouldn't be reading this book right now. You're in a rut, a slump, and you're beginning to think that nothing—or nobody—will ever be able to help you to eat right, exercise effectively, and live a long, healthy life.

But that just isn't so. In fact, we each have within ourselves an incredibly powerful tool to help us live up to our full potential. That's right; the one thing you need to change your life forever is waiting right inside of you, just waiting for you to unlock the door to a way of life few discover, but all can enjoy.

What is that one thing, the one secret the fad diets fail to consider?

The power of the mind.

This may sound like some New Age mumbo-jumbo, but stay with me a moment here. After all, the mind controls every facet of the human body. Without your mind, your body would cease to function; without your mind, you wouldn't be able to read this book because you wouldn't be able to comprehend the words, and you wouldn't be able to exercise because you wouldn't be able to control your muscles. Ultimately, without the mind, the body will falter. Likewise, without the mind any attempt to improve, condition, train, hone, or slim the body will falter as well. Leaving the mind out of the fitness equation is like leaving a vital ingredient out of your favorite recipes. You may see results, but the finished dish just won't taste quite right.

So, the logical solution to exercise and diet is to have a program that addresses the needs of the mind and body together, as one. Working on the physical without concentrating on the mental will not only lessen the results of any fitness or diet regimen, but it will also lessen your willpower to continue the regimen in the first place.

Although the *Mind Over Muscle* principles are unique, they are not necessarily new. Many of the techniques you'll read about here have actually been around for centuries. You may even be familiar with some of them—you may, for instance, have tried meditation in order to reduce stress or used guided imagery to help you get over a phobia. And if you've ever tried yoga or Pilates—or used the Zone-Tone Technique featured in my bestselling fitness books, *The Body Sculpting Bible* series—then you've gotten a taste of how the mind and body can work together. Everyone from Deepak Chopra to Oprah Winfrey has discovered the power of the mind.

The Zone-Tone Technique (which you'll also find in this book) is a simple but very powerful and extremely successful method that works by focusing the mind's intent (Zone) on specific muscles throughout the body (Tone), for more intense workouts and remarkable results. Although I was firmly convinced of the Zone-Tone's effectiveness, even I was surprised by the incredible feedback I got from hundreds of thousands of readers.

Spurred in part by these loyal and enthusiastic readers and in part by my own interest in expanding my brain capacity, I began to research other techniques to help harness the power of the mind. You may have heard the factoid that humans only use about 10% of the brain's potential. I wanted to know why, and I wanted to find out if I could tap into the other 90% of the brain's potential.

After over a decade of research, reading countless books, interviewing top experts, and conducting hands-on experiments, I discovered a treasure trove of techniques to tap into the incredible power that lies within all of us. Some, like meditation, are ancient spiritual practices that scientists are just now beginning to understand; the exciting fields of quantum physics, neurology, and molecular biology, among others, have fostered an understanding of how thinking physically affects the neurons in our brain, which in turn affects the muscles those neurons control.

The main purpose of this book is to teach you how to use these very powerful techniques that will truly enhance your body's ability to transform physically. Our bodies are magical, marvelous, amazing creations; they can run for miles and lift more pounds than we ever imagined. The muscles can heal and repair, weight can be lost, and it takes much less food than we think we need to run the human body efficiently and purposefully. It is not the physical that fails us when we cheat on our diets or let our gym memberships lapse. Most times it is a lack of mental training—not physical stamina or endurance—that actually causes a person to abandon a workout and dieting regimen.

This is a book about change; real, lasting, active, revolutionary change. It's a book about new ideas based on old principles, and old dogs learning new tricks. It's not your grandmother's diet book or even your father's bodybuilding book; far from it. The *Mind Over Muscle* principles are very powerful and very real. They're also very easy and accessible to all. If you give them a chance, they will help you reach your goal.

I've worked very hard to create a comprehensive resource that could just be the very last book on health, nutrition, and exercise you own. (Except for the sequel, of course!) I know we're all busy; I know your time is precious. So is mine. So I've created a one-stop book that has it all: fitness, diet, energy. How did I do it? How did I pack all that stuff in here? How can a book with fewer than 300 pages possibly contain everything you'll ever need to look better, live longer, and feel better?

Simple: this is the first fitness book to tone your mind as well as your muscles. Since we're approaching the fitness spectrum from the head down—literally—I will give you not just the techniques you'll need to firm muscles or lose weight, but the mental tools you'll need to *enjoy* firming muscles and staying fit.

That's right; you can enjoy fitness because once you tap into the mind's awesome power for controlling the body you'll get addicted to the positive, healthful, youthful feelings that are part and parcel of the mind-body connection. You'll want to feel this way every day for the rest of your life because, for the very first time, all of you will benefit: mind, body, and soul.

A key element of this book is that no matter where you fall on the fitness scale it will work for you. Why? Because it offers program options for three main levels of fitness: beginner, intermediate, and advanced, and makes the mind the predominant "muscle" we are exercising. This holistic premise makes this the right book for you now, no matter how old you are or where you fall on the fitness spectrum.

If there is just one thing I want to mention before you begin your journey through *Mind Over Muscle*, it is this: have an open mind! The things that you are about to read may seem far-fetched at first and will most likely be very new to you, but hang on. According to a recent study by Harvard researchers Dr. Ellen Langer and Alia J. Crum, people who think they're getting a good workout obtain more benefits than those who perform the same activities but don't believe they are exercising. "It is clear," they write, "that health is significantly affected by mindset.

In this program I will show you how to attack your weight loss and physical fitness deficiencies by utilizing a two-pronged approach. The first prong is an introduction of the mental techniques that will help strengthen the mind and your willpower. The second prong includes a complete 6 to 10 week exercise routine that will help you combine the mental and physical exercises and actually have fun exercising.

There will be no missing ingredient in this recipe. On the following pages I have provided all you'll need—in one easy resource—to attain your ultimate fitness goals. All you have to do is follow my advice, stay true to your program, set realistic goals, and above all remember one driving factor behind this revolutionary new program: the mind really *does* matter!

PART ONE:

The Mind

The program you're about to embark on is holistic—it encompasses all the aspects you will need to attain any and all of your fitness goals, be they ambitious or just testing the waters. It includes weight and cardiovascular training, nutrition, supplementation, rest and recuperation, and, most importantly, the proper mindset and mental training. I don't want you to come away from this experience only partially prepared; I want you to have everything you need to create your greatest body ever—in the shortest amount of time—right here between these covers. You won't have to wait for the sequel to get to the "good stuff." In fact, the "good stuff" starts right here, right now.

For our purposes, the mind is a muscle you will need to train, tap into, and access. You may not be able to see your mind bulge like a bicep, but to attain the body you've always wanted in the quickest amount of time—and maintain the results for the long-term—you must tap into those parts of your brain you never knew existed.

Don't get me wrong; I'm not saying you can just sit there and "mind-meld" yourself into the perfect human specimen. Just like muscles work in concert, so too does the mind-body connection. You need to work your body and your mind together. This is a holistic approach. We're going from top to bottom and back again, until you see a total body workout is really just that: exercise for the total body. So, in this section, get ready to start at the top.

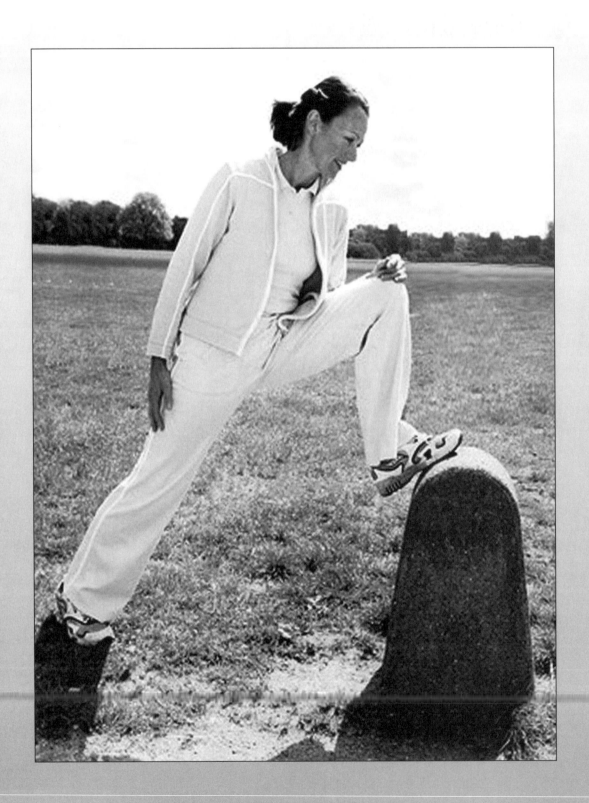

Chapter 1:

The Five Essential Stages

Message to reader: Read and re-read this section!

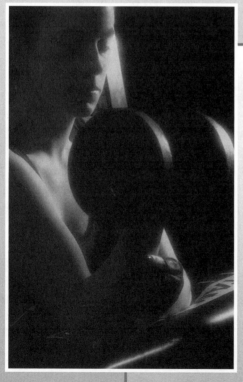

Every program begins with a solid foundation, and in this chapter, I will introduce you to the building blocks of the *Mind Over Muscle* program. These are more than mere suggestions to warm up before exercising or drink more water; these are the active, specific, and proven foundations for your personal fitness plan. These are the Five Essential Stages:

1ST STAGE: Relaxation

2ND STAGE: Breathing

3RD STAGE: Intention

4TH STAGE: Focus

5TH STAGE: Conviction

So What Is the Mind-Muscle Connection?

For nearly three decades, the mind-body field has gradually moved beyond the notion of segmented biological systems—i.e. the "pieces-parts," instead of the sum of the parts—but the idea of a mind-muscle connection is really not new. In the fourth century B.C., Hippocrates, a Greek philosopher educated and trained in the area of medicine, was the first to separate medicine from religion, and disease from supernatural explanations. He equated health to a harmonious balance of the mind, body, and the environment (Goleman and Gurin).

In the 1960s, a doctor named Herbert Benson opened a cardiac practice and often saw patients with elevated levels of hypertension. He hypothesized that it was the stress, brought on by the thinking in their mind, which was causing the hypertension. In order to test this theory, Dr. Benson went back to Harvard Medical School to perform some tests. Dr. Benson states that he "trained squirrel monkeys to either raise or lower blood pressure using operant conditioning technology. We found that the monkeys that were 'rewarded' for higher blood pressure went on to develop hypertension, due to their own behaviors" (Benson). The "reward" part of his study was most interesting because it shows how Dr. Benson conditioned the monkeys to have higher blood pressure. You can also influence your body through your thinking (mind). You can train your mind to affect the abilities of your body and your muscles to push further than you believe they can.

Later, Dr. Benson decided to run some tests on people who practiced meditation exercises (similar to those you'll find in this book). Dr. Benson found that through the simple act of changing their thought patterns, the subjects experienced decreases in their metabolism, breathing rate and brain wave frequency. He called these changes the "relaxation response."

Dr. Benson's final finding was that the relaxation techniques associated with his mind-body theory can also help in the healing process. He found that clinical studies over the years have shown the effectiveness of interventions on a wide range of medical problems caused (or made worse by) stress, such as hypertension, cardiac arrhythmias, pain, insomnia, allergies, repetitive stress injury and infertility, among many others (Benson). His findings were of great importance, not only to science but to every person who wanted to improve his or her life.

Mind-body connections don't just occur in laboratories; they are all around us. The discomfort associated with public speaking or the way a person's face may turn red or sweat when embarrassed are examples of a strong mind-body connection (Gandee, Knierim, and Mclittle-Marino). Your perception and mental evaluation of stimuli determines the degree of the mind-body response you experience. Your mental attitude toward potentially negative experiences is the key to stress management (Gandee, Knierim, and Mclittle-Marino).

When you are stressed and in a negative mood, your brain tells the body to release stress hormones even when the body does not really need them. There are two groups of stress hormones—catecholamines, including adrenaline and noradrenaline, increase heart rate and blood pressure; corcosteroids, including cortisone and cortisol, lead to nerve cell loss (Gandee, Knierim, and Mclittle-Marino).

How Can the Mind-Muscle Connection Help Me When I Work Out?

The mind-muscle connection is simply the combination of physical exercise executed with a profound, inwardly directed focus. This "inward focus" shouldn't conjure up images of aromatherapy candles and crystal balls; it can be more basically defined as paying greater attention (mind) to what is being experienced by the muscles and breath (body).

Now, we've all been told to "focus on our breathing" or "feel the burn" while we're working out. That's one kind of focus, but not *entirely* inward. What we're talking about here is a more centered approach to the entire process: what you're eating, why you're eating it, while you're driving to the gym or walking downstairs to your rowing machine, how you breathe before, during, and after exercise. That's what holistic means: the whole sum of your parts.

Like most Americans, you've probably been concentrating on your pieces-parts for most of your fitness life; a thigh here or a tummy there, a bicep here or a quadricep there. And it's worked. Don't get me wrong, I've written entire books on abs alone, and they've helped me and thousands of readers to spot-check that particular part of our bodies.

The mind-body connection, this holistic approach, works better—and faster—because we don't just see how having better abs will help us fit into our favorite pair of jeans again or look good for bikini season; it helps us see how having better abs affects our posture, metabolism, self-confidence, rate of breathing, and even our quality of sleep, work, and play.

This "inward focus," this concentration, leads to the contemplative state often attributed to mind-body practices. It's more than just a runner's high or the good feeling you get driving home from the gym. In fact, the best way to explain the mind-body connection is to suggest that your runner's high, that euphoric feeling which results when the mind and body are plugged into each other, can last all day, *every* day.

That's our goal for you. To guide you toward the discovery of this mind-body connection within yourself, I begin with the Five Essential Stages of the *Mind Over Muscle* holistic program.

1st STAGE:
Relaxation

Relaxation techniques are often perceived as passive, inactive ways of releasing all tension from muscles. Yet along with passive relaxation techniques for resting and recuperating after experiencing stress, active relaxation techniques can help people function in a relaxed and effective manner even during stressful or strenuous activity. It has been scientifically proven that functioning in a more relaxed manner not only prevents stress but also improves different kinds of performance.

If the *Mind Over Muscle* program is a puzzle, relaxation is the time you spend laying out the pieces, moving them around, seeing which ones might fit where, and getting yourself comfortable for the puzzle session to come. In the right, relaxed frame of mind, your pieces go together more quickly, easily, and smoothly because you're prepared to see the parts, the sum of the parts, and the big picture.

Right about now you're probably asking yourself, "Why relax before we even begin to exert ourselves? I thought I was going to learn how to get in better shape, not how to relax!?!" And you'd be right; this is a very good question! But remember what I said in the introduction about keeping an open mind? Well, here is where that really comes in handy.

The idea here is that by relaxing, we fully ready our minds and bodies for the upcoming workout. Relaxing allows us to become receptive to the exercise; to visualize the results we hope to achieve.

When was the last time you finished your workout and realized that it was the absolute best workout of your life? I'm not just talking about a few endorphins giving you a "workout high" that fades by the time you've showered and changed.

I'm talking about an invigorating, reviving, head-to-toe feeling that made this workout the absolute best you've ever experienced. It happens. Some days are better than others. We're better rested, in a better mood, our bodies feel looser, our muscles more responsive and less resistant, we feel plugged in from the moment we begin until our very last rep. Unfortunately, the many people who have experienced that feeling—myself included—have had a very difficult time trying to duplicate and achieve that very same satisfied feeling on a consistent basis.

The next day we seek that perfect workout, yet it eludes us. Traffic is heavier, we're more tired, the gym's more crowded, we're just not "feeling it." Why? What's the difference between Monday's workout and Wednesday's?

Here's the problem: you most probably achieved that "perfect workout" because for once in your life you were "fully there." It can be very difficult to fully focus on our true objective: exercising. We tend to allow other things, like the music on the stereo or the really buff guy next to

us or the afternoon meeting we're headed to after the gym, distract our ability to fully focus. We soldier through the reps, the sets, the miles, the laps, but we're not getting the full benefit out of them because we're in pieces-parts mode.

When you learn to fully relax the mind and body from outside influences, your best workout will be your next workout and every workout after that will exceed the last, living up to and surpassing your greatest expectation and fulfillment. You *will* create your greatest body ever—in the shortest amount of time—because every workout will be better than the last.

The ability to voluntarily relax is the first step to controlling your mind. The process of relaxation results in a sense of mind-body integration that allows a person to control emotions, anxiety, and even physiological functions, which collectively constitute "pressure." Moreover, relaxation allows the appropriate part of the brain, the right brain, to perform some of the complex skills without interference from the left brain.

The two major relaxation techniques are muscle-to-mind and mind-to-muscle. The goal of muscle-to-mind relaxation is to train the muscles to be sensitive to any tension and to reach an ability to release that tension. This technique is based on the belief that an anxious, fearful mind cannot exist in a relaxed body. Therefore, relaxing the muscles relaxes the mind.

EXERCISE:
Mind-to-Muscle Relaxation

Step 1: Detach . . . from the "white" noise of your day: Background stimuli such as honking horns, people talking on phones, music, or other people's conversations can distract us from true relaxation. You must learn to detach from this "white noise," to unplug yourself from the outside stressors of the world. To accomplish this difficult task, pick one word, a mantra if you will, and repeat it over and over until it becomes your sole focus. I usually choose a word like "relax" or "soothe" to keep my mind oriented to its ultimate goal. Repeat it over and over again until you find yourself starting to relax, then:

Step 2: Decide . . . that relaxation is a priority: You can't passively relax, you must *actively* relax. While this may sound like a contradiction in terms, we must shift our idea of relaxation as something ineffectual and lazy to something dynamic and beneficial. The only way to do so is to make relaxation a priority, not a luxury.

Step 3: Direct . . . your sole attention to quieting your mind: Free yourself to relax; give your mind permission to quiet itself from the concerns, fears, and doubts of your day. You can typically achieve this state while stretching, driving to the gym, or lacing up your running shoes. Make relaxing a habit; direct yourself to relax at the same time each day, or during the same routine.

EXERCISE:
Muscle-to-Mind ("Sense, Then Tense") Relaxation

The following relaxation technique will help you to become more familiar with the various muscles of your body. We will begin with the muscles of the lower body and move up to the shoulders, isometrically contracting (that is, tightening the muscle without moving it) and then relaxing each one. As you do this, you may feel muscles in your body that you've never felt before. There is no better way to fully master your ability to control your muscles, which will inevitably make your workouts the absolute best they've ever been.

Very Important: Isometric exercise can increase blood pressure and heart rate to levels that would be danger-

ous for anyone with undiagnosed cardiac problems. If you have—or are not sure if you are prone to—such health ailments, consult with your physician before beginning this technique! If your muscles cramp, don't panic and give up; simply relax, wait a little while and then begin again. Remember to breathe deeply throughout the exercise.

Step 1: Please begin by lying down on your back, making sure that you are in a very comfortable position.

Step 2: We begin with the shin muscle, located on the front portion of the lower leg, between the top of your foot and just below the kneecap. With the legs fully extended and relaxed, flex your feet and toes up toward your knees, while contracting the muscles of the front shin. Hold the contraction for at least 10 seconds, tensing the muscle group as tightly as you can, then relax completely.

Step 3: Next we move to the calf muscles, located on the back of your leg between the heel and behind the kneecap. To engage the calf muscles, flex your feet and push your toes away from you (imagine yourself on tiptoe), while contracting the muscles of the calf. Curling the toes up will increase the contraction of the calf muscle. Hold the contraction for at least 10 seconds, tensing the muscle group as tightly as you can, then relax completely.

Step 4: Now we're on to the quadricep muscles of the front thigh, located between the top of the kneecap and just below the front portion of your hips. To engage the quadricep muscles, keep your legs fully extended and lock out the knee. This should help you feel those muscles contracting, and is a key part of this exercise. Hold the contraction for at least 10 seconds, tensing the muscle group as tightly as you can, then relax completely.

Step 5: Next are the hamstring muscles, positioned directly behind the quadriceps and located between the back of the knee and just below the crease of the buttocks. To engage the hamstring muscles, slightly bend the knees and without moving the knee joint, contract the hamstring. It might help to think of the hamstring muscles as the biceps of your legs, so you'd hold them tight the same way you would flex your bicep. Hold the contraction for at least 10 seconds, tensing the muscle group as tightly as you can, then relax completely.

Step 6: Now we move directly up to the gluteal or butt muscles. To engage these muscles, simply squeeze your cheeks together and feel the muscles actually push the center of your body slightly off the bed or floor. This is how you'll know they're working. Hold the contraction for at least 10 seconds, tensing the muscle group as tightly as you can, then relax completely

Step 7: Let's move back to the front of the body, to the abdominal muscles. This muscle group is located between the top of your pelvis and all the way up to just below your chest muscles. To engage the abdominal muscles, think about what happens when you cough. When you cough, your body naturally reacts by tensing your abdominal muscles. To engage these muscles without having to cough, forcefully attempt to exhale without allowing the air to escape your lungs and simultaneously press your lower back into the floor. This will automatically engage the abdominal muscles. Please do not hold your breath for more than a few seconds. If you have any type of high blood pressure or contra-indicative health concerns, please avoid this particular step altogether. Hold the contraction for at least 10 seconds, tensing the muscle group as tightly as you can, then relax completely.

Step 8: The next set of muscles are the lower back muscles, known as the erector spinae muscles, located just above the butt and up to the mid-back. The best way to contract these muscles is by creating a more pronounced curve in your lower lumbar back region. To do this most efficiently, it will help to stick out your chest and butt at the same time. This very subtle movement will help to contract these sometimes challenging muscles. Hold the contraction for at least 10 seconds, tensing the muscle group as tightly as you can, then relax completely.

Step 9: Now we move to the mid- and outer back muscles, known as the latissimus dorsi muscles or "lats." To engage these muscles, bring your shoulders back and imagine them touching each other behind you. Simultaneously press your shoulder blades into the floor. Hold the contraction for at least 10 seconds, tensing the muscle group as tightly as you can, then relax completely.

Step 10: Now let's go back to the front of the body, to the chest muscles, also known as the pectoral muscles or "pecs." To contract these muscles, bring your shoulders toward each other, but don't allow them to really move. Inhibiting the actual shoulders from moving toward each other will help to engage the chest muscles. Hold the contraction for at least 10 seconds, tensing the muscle group as tightly as you can, then relax completely.

Step 11: On to the shoulders. The shoulders are perhaps the most difficult muscles to contract. As you did in the previous step, bring your shoulders toward each other, but don't allow them to really move. Or try pressing the shoulder blades back into the floor. This time, think about tensing all of your shoulder muscles. Hold the contraction for at least 10 seconds, tensing the muscle group as tightly as you can, then relax completely.

Step 12: Finally we reach the trapezius, or upper shoulder, muscles. These muscles are located at the base of the neck and move down to the upper back region. To engage these muscles, first bring the shoulder blades back, as you've done before but focus on the trapezius muscles. Hold the contraction for at least 10 seconds, tensing the muscle group as tightly as you can, then relax completely.

Step 13: Now, still working on the trapezius muscles, shrug your shoulders up toward your ears and hold. In other words, pull the top of your shoulders up as high as you can and hold. Hold the contraction for at least 10 seconds, tensing the muscle group as tightly as you can, then relax completely.

Step 14: Once you have worked your way up to your shoulders, contract your whole body in unison, hold for 10 seconds, then relax.

2nd STAGE:
Breathing

Breathing can either be spontaneous and natural, an organic response to the moment, or it can be habitual, mechanical, and reactive. In other words, we either allow our breathing to control us, or we learn to effectively and powerfully control our breathing.

Breathing is the ultimate mind-body disconnect. We do it automatically, subconsciously, all day long, without ever being "fully there." Our mind (the brain) tells our body (the lungs) to breathe all day long, without us ever doing anything active or focused about it.

Talk about neglecting one of our body's most powerful tools. Breathing is, without question, one of your best tools when it comes to increasing athletic performance, mood, mindset, health and, yes, even the look of your physique. Did you know that every day we take between 16,000 and 23,000 breaths? We're already conditioned to breathe, so why not accentuate this dormant power system so that it works to our advantage?

The benefits associated with voluntary breathing techniques didn't truly penetrate the mainstream fitness and health market until yoga first became popular. Unfortunately, it was often dismissed by many as "hokey," New Age, or metaphysical. As time has proven, however, the physical benefits of yoga are significant and long-lasting, and we have much to learn from this lesson.

Let's examine breathing from a health standpoint. When you are feeling sick, have you ever noticed how your breathing is affected? Whether it is a cold, flu, or a bronchial infection, your illness is often accompanied by shallow, short or irregular breathing. When you experience these short and restricted irregular breaths, you will most often experience a feeling of being lethargic and exhausted. On the other hand, if you have ever experienced taking very fast or uncontrolled deep breaths, such as during great stress or even panic, it can result in feeling dizzy or lightheaded. In other words, our breathing can most definitely control our body.

Breathing can also control the mind. Haven't you ever seen a person who was really nervous, uptight or embarrassed, taking very deep and methodical breaths? They are actually helping to calm their minds through the use of deep breathing techniques. "Energized breathing," or taking quick but measured breaths, actually helps to dispel negative and depressive moods by releasing the neurotransmitters serotonin, norepinephrine, and dopamine, the chemicals that help regulate your energy and emotion (Thayer).

In exercising, you are putting your body through what basically amounts to a "planned attack." Breathing correctly before, during, and after exercising will help control stress. In order to give your body the energy it needs while you exercise, breathe in through the nose and out through the mouth. If you breathe only through your mouth, you may reach a point where your lungs are fighting for every breath. Learning to breathe in through your nose and out your mouth is the first step to effective controlled and energized breathing.

Breathing is actually the only visceral (autonomic) function that we can consciously control. That might not seem like a great fitness fact, but I assure you, it is. We don't want to be controlled, so here's how to get in control.

EXERCISE:
Breathing for Relaxation
(Belly Breathing)

The ability to breathe deeply through the diaphragm, sometimes called "belly breathing," is an integral part of deep relaxation.

Step 1: The in-breath, which you'll do in three steps, should last for a count of 5. First, fill the lower third of your lungs by forcing the diaphragm down and therefore raising the abdomen. Then, fill the middle third of your lungs by expanding the lower part of the chest cavity. Finally, fill the upper third of your lungs after raising the shoulders and chest slightly.

Step 2: Empty your lungs in reverse order: first, the upper third, then the middle, and finally the lower third. The out-breath should last for a count of 6. This 5:6 ratio seems to be a simple yet powerful way you can induce a relaxed state at will.

Step 3: Continue the process for at least 2 minutes, or 10 breaths.

EXERCISE:
Breathing for Exercise

It is vital that you develop a good breathing rhythm as you work out. Not only will it relax you, but it will help keep you focused. Try to avoid being too dramatic with your breathing. I've seen trainers tell their clients to "Breathe! Breathe! Breathe!" and the next thing you know, their client is hyperventilating. Breathe naturally and easily. Whether you're a gym rat or first-time exercise newbie, here is a quick recap of how breathing is typically taught at the gym:

Step 1: As you begin the positive portion of an exercise (pressing the weight up while doing a bench press, for instance), exhale. Exhaling during the exertion allows the body to get rid of (expel) stagnant oxygen, thus giving you the ability to once again take a deeper breath.

Step 2: Inhale when you descend to the negative portion of the repetition (in the bench press example, this is when you lower the bar toward your chest). Inhaling deeply before each exertion of a repetition allows the muscles to have maximum oxygen for peak performance and safety.

EXERCISE:
Breathing for the Rest
of the Time (Dog Breath)

Here is a breathing exercise that will help calm your mind in tense or stressful moments. It will also raise your metabolism, causing your body to feel warm as it burns more calories.

Step 1: Lie down on your bed or a clear space on the floor.

Step 2: Breathe rapidly through your mouth, panting like a dog. Take 20 quick breaths in this manner.

Step 3: Now breathe slowly and deeply through your nose 20 times.

Step 4: Return to panting for 20 breaths, then another set of 20 slow, deep breaths.

Step 5: Repeat this pattern until your mind becomes relaxed and you feel a warm sensation throughout your body.

3rd STAGE:
Intention

What's so critical about your intention is that it guides your entire fitness program. It's not just your sense of purpose for working out; it IS your purpose for working out. It's the reason you get out of bed in the morning, lace those running shoes, and head out for that jog. It's the reason you pay those gym fees and put up with the crowds and lift those weights.

Intention becomes the reason why we take the pieces-parts of our fitness puzzle out, move them around, and put them together. It's why we sit down to our puzzle table in the first place and what keeps us there when the pieces don't fit or the grooves don't mesh. It's also what makes us reach for another puzzle as soon as the first one is finished. Without intention, our puzzle pieces—i.e., our fitness goals—stay moldy and musty in their boxes, gathering dust with the rest of the good intentions we failed to follow through on.

I'll help you define your fitness goals in more detail in Chapter 2, but first ask yourself: What has brought you here? What is your exact reason for wanting to create a perfect physique? These may sound like dumb questions at this point, but it's of the utmost importance to discover exactly what it is you want from this program so that it

can become a powerhouse in helping you to achieve that intention.

We all think that strong muscles and proper nutrition are the backbone upon which your perfect body is built, and they're important, but your intentions and attitude are two of the most important factors when it comes to your decisions about exercising. In order to achieve success you must first decide what, exactly, you want to attain from it. Verbalize your intention and visualize it, picturing what you want in your mind and keeping that image firmly before you until your intention is brought to fruition.

What is it you intend to get out of this exercise program?

EXERCISE:
Discovering Desire, Belief,
and Acceptance

The following exercise will help you discover the truth behind your desire, the limits of your belief, and the level of your acceptance.

Step 1: Write down one of your personal goals, such as "losing weight," "joining a gym," or "walking 3 miles a week." _____

_____

_____

Step 2: Now write down the feeling you will have once you attain that goal. Try to pick a single word to describe the feeling, such as confidence, longevity, or healthfulness. _____

_____

That feeling is your *real* goal, or intention.

Now let's take this a little bit further:

Step 3: Desire: What, exactly, do you want to achieve?

_____

_____

_____

Step 4: Belief: Do you truly believe you can have what you desire?

_____

_____

_____

Step 5: Acceptance: What commitment is required to achieve that desire?

_____

_____

_____

Step 6: Alignment: Do your desires, beliefs, and commitment level match your intent for following this program?

_____

_____

_____

EXERCISE:
Determining Intentions

Complete the following sentences to help define your intention and direction for this program:

I intend to look like _____

_____

_____

I intend to feel like _____

_____

_____

I intend to be able to _____

_____

_____

I intend to have _____

_____

_____

The beauty of these exercises is that they reveal to people that their goals might not really be aligned with their true intentions. If people focused more on the end result of happiness, security, and financial freedom, perhaps they could reach their goals on many different levels and in many different ways, rather than just "hoping for a million dollars," which may be a bit far-fetched . . . or a long time coming.

4th STAGE:
Focus

Focus is the key to being fully there while you exercise; focus is the glue that holds the pieces-parts together and gives us our holistic sum of our parts. None of these Essential Stages is more important than the next—in other words, they're not ranked in any specific order—but I can't stress strongly enough how important it is to focus when you're exercising.

When you think of the word "focus," you probably think it means simply concentrating on something and, in a broad sense, you'd be right. But here, I define focus as the ability to perform under all circumstances, regardless of the possible distractions and negative influences around you. Your ability to concentrate during exercise and mentally remain within the present moment—to be fully there—is vital if you want your fitness goals to be reached quickly. Relaxation, as we saw in Stage 1, is the first step to tuning out distractions and being fully there. Then, focus hones in like a razor-sharp thought on the finite and specific task we are doing at that moment.

When you are doing a bicep curl, for instance, focus on how your arms are working. Feel your muscles contract and imagine them getting leaner and stronger as your body progresses toward its ultimate state of muscular fitness. This is not the same as visualization, in which you imagine what the future will entail. Do not focus on the future, but on the present moment. You can focus on your muscles while you are not exercising as well. When you are warming up, imagine your muscles becoming more agile; when you are resting, imagine your muscles healing themselves and becoming stronger. Focus on the muscles and the body will do the rest.

This real, concentrated, clear, and precise focus, where you are locked in and fully engaged during a particular task, is essential for achieving peak performance in any endeavor, but particularly when it comes to the mind-body connection. While we all slip into a rut when tasks are repeated over and over again—think how routine it can be to check your email at work or cook dinner at home—peak performance can only be obtained when you remain focused during every workout, every day. Switching in and out of concentration—losing focus—will hold you back from achieving your ultimate fitness goals.

Focus can feel almost euphoric, as time can quickly pass by without your being aware of its passing. You've heard the saying, "Time flies when you're having fun." Well, the same applies here! Time and outside influences will go on doing what they do best—pass you by—while you do what you do best: train with an effortless mindset and passion.

Dr. Mihaly Csikszentmihaly, a psychologist at the University of Chicago, calls this phenomenon "flow." His studies involved athletes of all types cyclists, video gamers, soccer players, rock climbers—an eclectic mix of people who despite outward appearances had one thing in common: they loved what they did and had to concentrate fully to achieve their peak performance. He found that "when people become fully absorbed in an activity, they reach a state of flow."(Csikszentmihaly) Now,

this is where I believe the subtitle of this book, "The Effortless Way to a Perfect Body," makes absolutely perfect sense. When you love doing something, it's no longer considered work; it becomes a pleasurable act and with pleasure comes a combination of timelessness, passion, fun, and results.

EXERCISE:
Focus on Exercise

Step 1: Concentrate on the specific exercise that you are about to do. Focus on the specific muscles you intend to isolate. Think about how much weight you intend to lift and how many repetitions you must perform.

Step 2: Now hone in on your feelings and thoughts. You will experience changes from one workout to the next. You might be feeling down one day and up the next, you might have little energy one day and lots the next. Without forcing it, focus your thoughts on feeling ready and interested in your exercise.

Step 3: Now hone in on your action. As you perform the exercise, focus on what your muscles are doing and feel them growing stronger and leaner.

5th STAGE:
Conviction

Our fifth and final Essential Stage, conviction, can best be defined as an unshakable belief in something without need for proof or evidence. When you demonstrate conviction in these principles, when you believe in them and adhere to them, I want you to know without a shadow of a doubt that you will receive the results you expect.

If focus is the glue that holds all five of these Essentials together, then conviction is the groove that allows all five pieces to fit together. With conviction, you believe in your success, envision the results, and dedicate yourself fully to a repeated pattern of practices—exercise, eating right, sleeping better, focusing—to achieve those results.

Many people spend months, if not years, thinking about how they would one day love to begin an exercise regimen. We buy books, videos, more books, more videos, and have enough "free gym trial" coupons to use as dusty bookmarks for all those dusty exercise and fitness books! It's human nature; inspiration is fleeting and life gets in the way. As a result, the days pass by and your inspiration becomes yet another moment suspended—and passed by—in time.

So what do we do? How do we finally take the first step to everlasting physical change? Well, we start from where we are. We don't have to be at our ideal weight to walk into a gym. We don't have to look like a personal trainer to jog, or even walk, around the block.

We start small, we start slow, and we start . . . where . . . we . . . are. We don't wait until tomorrow because that will just lead to more excuses and, frankly, another tomorrow. We don't wait until that new gym down the street finishes construction or until our skin clears up; we decide, we commit, and we do so with conviction. It is often said that "a journey of a thousand miles begins with a single footstep." This is your journey; this is your first step.

Trust me, all it takes is that very first step, because once you begin to see physical changes to your body and feel the extraordinary additional benefits that accompany the *Mind Over Muscle* holistic program, you will not want to stop.

Unfortunately, along the way, you will most likely encounter obstacles, such as temptation, stubbornness, laziness, boredom and just plain old life getting in the middle of it all.

There might be times when you cheat on your diet, miss a few workouts, sustain an injury, or feel like you're not achieving results. A setback or challenge like this can discourage you from returning to exercise again.

But don't give up: the "pot of gold" or "reaping of results" is just around the corner. Reaching your fitness goals is inevitable when you consistently follow a proven plan of action. This is the true meaning of conviction; believing without seeing, continuing to act in a committed path when results aren't immediately visible.

Success won't come over-night; results won't happen in a day. Don't give up because you look like your old self one day and don't look like an Adonis or Aphrodite the next. We don't plant a tree on Sunday and dig up the seeds on Friday because it's not big enough for our tree fort yet. So why should we abandon our plans for a better, healthier, happier body just because we hit the wall or face a plateau when we were just starting to build some momentum?

With conviction, results happen because you *believe* they will happen…

EXERCISE:
Determining Your Conviction

Step 1: To determine your firm convictions, write down a statement, make it a paragraph, about why you're beginning on this *Mind Over Muscle* quest. It should read something like this:

> *I believe that it is time to change my life and make better use of my time. I want to have a better, stronger appearance because I think it is time for me to start looking better and feeling better. I'm not getting any younger, and I know that if I don't start this program now I will spend another year wishing I had.*

Step 2: Now, strike through all the fat; erase or scribble out all the words that don't stand for a distinct belief (or conviction). For instance, once I cut the fat from my statement I was left with two strong convictions:

1. *I believe that it is time to change my life.*

2. *I know that if I don't start this program now I will spend another year wishing I had.*

EXERCISE:
Repeating Your Conviction

How do you keep your conviction at the forefront of your thinking? It is very simple and involves a basic meditation technique of repeating a phrase, or mantra. This exercise keeps your conviction in your mind at all times and helps you zero in on your conviction and believe that your conviction is possible to achieve.

Step 1: Think of one simple word or phrase that reflects your convictions. I use the phrase "No problem." You might even choose the word "conviction"—just the word itself conjures up images of strength and belief.

Step 2: Repeat this phrase 10 times in your head (or out loud if you prefer). Every time you repeat these words keep thinking of your overall goal, and you will soon associate your overall goal as being "no problem" to achieve. Repeat this phrase 10 times before your exercises, in between exercises (between sets, for instance), and once again after your exercises. You can even do this exercise in the shower. You can repeat the phrase and let the water hit your head and almost get into a meditation type of state.

EXERCISE:
Integrating Your Conviction with Your Life

Step 1: Post a note on the mirror where you remind yourself of the exercise program you are currently working in. The reminder must be posted in a location that you will always see. The goal here is to make yourself feel guilty if you skip a day of working out.

Step 2: Once you see the reminder visualize what you must do for that day. Are you working arms or legs? Are you doing some cardio exercise? Once you decide what the goal is for the day, your next step is to accept the time it will take to complete the goal for that day and accept the fact that your program is basically, at this point, a job—a job you love. You must show up and you must perform. It is mandatory if you want to succeed.

By performing this conviction exercise everyday, your program will become a routine, something that is integrated into your life. You will soon establish the fact that you *must* go work out; that is conviction. Your results will cause you to want to go more and more and the conviction will become ingrained in your mind and your life.

Bringing It All Together

I've found that, for many of my clients, issues arise during a drastic life change. After all, seeking perfection isn't easy. However, writing out their "problem of the day" helps them work through it. In the back of this book you will find my *Mind Over Muscle* Journal. It's quite painless, really. All the lines are there, and all you simply need to do is focus on one problem at a time. Writing can be beneficial, even if it's about weight machines or leotards!

Here is a place where the mind-body connection can really gel for you. Actively thinking about the processes involved in exercise, nutrition, supplementation, etc., will force you to focus, to be "fully there." Writing is a centering exercise; choose a time of day or night that works best for you and let 'er rip.

Write about your training, your trainer. Write about your eating habits, the good, the bad, the ugly, and the really, *really* ugly. Write about the pain, the release, the joy, the changes, the bad habits, the new habits, and how this experience is affecting you.

By being honest with yourself, by baring your soul, by challenging yourself to open up and invite the written word (the mind) to be a part of your sweat (the body) you will begin forging the mind-body connection for yourself.

Therefore, after going through the steps of relaxation, breathing, intention, focus, and conviction, visualize the overall master plan for yourself. What does it look like? What will you actively do about it? How will you effect change, every day, to bring these five *Mind Over Muscle* essentials into your daily life and create your greatest body ever—in the shortest amount of time? Here's an example for you:

DAY: Friday

Date: 03 / 08 / 2006

Problem of the Day: Today was an interesting day. I woke up feeling sore and unmotivated, in general. My first impulse was to "skip" today's workout, but then I remembered this journal so I thought I'd see if it really worked! Here goes:

Solution of the Day: I realized that the problem I was facing was mostly in my mind. Sure, I was sore, but by now I've seen enough flexing exercises that I could probably work those kinks out rather easily. Instead I focused on my mind, and looked for the best meditation exercise to really rewire my whole mental circuitry! I settled on the "sense then tense" method, and although it was a struggle kept through it until, a few minutes later, I really did feel a whole shift in my attitude. Not only was my mind re-booted, but by flexing/tensing my body I felt some of the soreness/stiffness go away as well. Next stop, the gym!

General Thoughts: I really, really, REALLY didn't want to exercise today. I know in the past I would have skipped working out today, no problem. I mean, in the grand scheme of things, who cares, right??? But this program urges us to be the best we've ever been before, and I'm really ready for a change. So, I did something I've never done before—stretched my mind as well as my muscles—and it really worked!

Chapter 2:

Mindful Preparation

Message to Reader: Use these daily tools and techniques to achieve the best possible outcome.

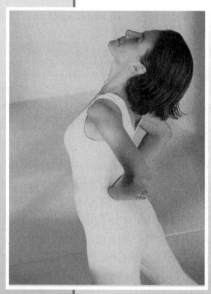

I have always believed that there is a time and a place for everything. What makes the difference when someone tries and tries to quit smoking, and finally does? How does one person lose 200 pounds or give up caffeine, or learn how to walk again after being in a terrible car accident, while others flounder in vain attempts for years? The answer, I've found, is surprisingly simple: people succeed when they're ready.

This section of the book, Mindful Preparation, is all about getting ready. Together, we're going to get you ready to have the body, health, and lifestyle that you've only dreamed about until now. In the rest of this chapter, I will give you six simple tools and techniques that you will want to use daily to help you excel in the *Mind Over Muscle* program. These are:

1. Goal Setting
2. Visualization
3. High Performance Meditation
4. Conscious Creation
5. Guided Imagery
6. Activation Sheet

Let's get started . .

STEP #1:
Goal Setting

Setting goals is one of the very best ways to help you achieve what you want. Goals provide us with mile-markers to let us know we're on our way to where we want to go. They motivate us by acknowledging our progress and giving us a sight on the horizon that we can see and hope to reach.

But goals don't motivate us if they don't have purpose and direction. If you're leaving Chicago on a road trip to New York, you don't set a goal of reaching the exit for Los Angeles. And if you do, you've delayed reaching your *real* destination.

So if our destination is to be slim and healthy so we can be more confident and alluring, we don't set a goal of watching 20 hours of TV each week. Like the glittery off ramp to LA, that kind of goal will only delay reaching our desired destination.

Setting a goal that overreaches our destination doesn't work, either. Deciding to run 20 miles a day, five days a week, is the kind of goal a marathon runner sets, not someone just looking to lose a few pounds. That kind of goal won't motivate us, because we know that it's further than we really want to go; it's like shooting to reach England when you want to get to New York.

People often choose goals without really thinking about their reasons for wanting to attain them. In other words, if you were to ask 8 out of 10 people what they'd want if they could have it "right now," they'd most often say something vague and automatic like, "A million dollars." However, it's often not the money that would bring most people satisfaction, but rather the feeling of security or freedom as a result of attaining the money.

So, in order to set goals that are motivating and meaningful, we turn to our intentions. In Chapter 1 we talked about intentions being the big reason for pursuing our exercise program.

Now, think back to your intentions, which you determined in Chapter 1. Once we know what we intend to get out of the program, it's time to set our goals.

Think of it this way: Goals are the plans we pencil in each day; intentions are the reason we pull out the pencil in the first place.

Goals have to take us in the direction of our intentions. For that reason, the goals we set must be very specific.

Don't just say, "Look better" or "Feel better." What, specifically, do you hope to accomplish on this program? Lose 10 pounds? Walk to Elm Street by 10:15 a.m. instead of 10:30? Fit back into those size 30-waist jeans (or size 5, for the ladies)?

Go a step further and include in your goal another specific result that stems from the first, such as "Fitting into those size 30-waist jeans makes me feel good. I'm more confident, and I can wear more stylish clothes so that I can impress the boss." Visualize the results of achieving your goals with as much punch and life as you can.

Begin with your long-term goals. Be very precise and provide as much detail as possible about your goal and how it will make you feel. (Use the *Mind Over Muscle* Activation Sheet as a guide to write this down.) Your long-term goals will no doubt seem pretty unattainable in the very beginning and that is to be expected. That's why we also develop short-term goals, which are smaller steps on the way to achieving our long-term goals. In fact, you'll also want to develop some medium-term goals, to help bridge the gap between your short- and long-term goals and give you some intermediate milestones to celebrate along the way. Together, the long-, medium-, and short-term goals will help to fuel your ability to reach physical perfection.

Your short-term goals should be analyzed at the

end of every week. It might seem like a very little time to notice any results at all, but the opposite is true. I want you to expect great changes to occur *every single day*. They might not manifest into the physical results that soon, but at the very least, your emotional and internal results should be expected, achieved, and celebrated on a daily basis.

Obviously, your short-term goals are going to be more easily attained than your long-term goals. However, by achieving each of your smaller short-term goals, you will be that much closer to realizing and achieving all of your long-term goals as well.

Finally, remember that sometimes what seems possible, or even reasonable, on Sunday night after dinner is a little harder to accomplish at 6 a.m. Monday morning. If your action plan proves to be too ambitious or unrealistic, modify it. After all, it won't be any good to you if it's just sitting on the fridge or in the back of this book. If you happen to miss your goals a little, don't get discouraged and don't punish yourself for it. Just set your new goals and be more determined in following your action plan so that you get there this time. If you messed up your plan for an entire day, let it go and get right back on track the following day.

You'll set your own personal goals on the *Mind Over Muscle* Activation Sheet at the end of this chapter, but I've also identified a short-, medium-, and long-term goal that every exerciser can use. The following exercises will help you get started in establishing your own, specific goals.

SHORT-TERM GOAL EXERCISE:
Decide what you want to do (and whether or not you think you are worth it!)

Step 1: With this goal you are simply deciding that you are important and that physical fitness should be a part

of your life. You will identify that there are some problem areas to work on and that you will, in fact, work on them. For this exercise you simply decide, once and for all, that you will join a workout program and will give it a determined try.

> **WARNING:** Don't skip this goal! It may seem like a no-brainer to commit to this exercise, but I can assure you that nothing could be further from the truth. Assumptions, I have found, are program killers. So many plans fail because we assume we're ready, we assume we've got all the necessary tools assembled at the ready, and we assume we don't need to set such an obvious goal.

The best part about this goal is that this is a very short-term goal. One might say it's a self-completing goal, because once you make the decision to at least try to change your life then the goal has already been attained. After you decide to change your life and body you can take charge in your life and feel a sense of accomplishment, because this is the step that people often falter with. They agree they need to change their life, but they do not start the process. Therefore they fail because their mind is not accepting any short-term goals to keep the momentum going.

MEDIUM-TERM GOAL EXERCISE:
Focus on feeling good and not too much on results

Step 1: Focus on how you feel after your first few workouts, instead of your waist size or the amount of weight you can lift or other results. Do you feel healthier? More energetic? Like you've accomplished a goal? Say to yourself: "I do not have dramatic physical results at the moment, but right now I am feeling the best I have felt in years, so I am going to stick with this exercise program until I can look as good as I feel!"

Step 2: Repeat this mantra: *I will feel better, I will have more energy, I will continue with the program.* Focusing on the lack of results will only lead to negative ideas about where you are headed and will contribute nothing to your overall well-being.

LONG-TERM GOAL EXERCISE:
The ultimate goal . . . finding your ideal look and physique

Step 1: Focus on your physique and not how much weight you are losing. Your goal is to have tight and toned muscles, not to have the scales register lower. Your goal is to have your clothes fit better, not to brag about how much weight you lost. Your goal is to be a healthy individual, not to try unhealthy behaviors in order to lose as much weight as possible. If weight loss is a priority for you, rest assured that the more muscle you build, the more that fat will burn. As your new physical self becomes apparent, as muscle replaces fat, weight loss will become less of an issue. Your goal is the ultimate physique and this is for the long-term.

> **WARNING:** *Do not give up!* Readjust your goals if you have to, reassess how you work out each day and what you may be doing right or wrong, don't stop the program altogether because you're not where you think you should be just yet. Just make another goal that is more attainable—and meet that new, revised goal. Once that goal is met, pursue the goal that you did not meet in the first place. By doing this you will not only keep your confidence, but you'll stay on the program and reach more goals than you ever thought imaginable.

STEP # 2:
Visualization

Visualization is a technique that is often used by professional athletes during practice or training, or just before the execution of the actual feat. The athlete imagines in her mind that she will perform the upcoming athletic feat flawlessly and with ease. When you do your visualizations, make your images as vivid and as real as possible. You must believe that what you are seeing, such as your victory in a race, has already happened. The subconscious mind cannot tell fantasy from reality and it will work hard to bring that recurrence into your reality. Remember, it's not enough to just have positive thoughts. You need to create **strong positive beliefs**. You must fully believe in yourself and your ability to accomplish all that you desire.

Okay, so maybe you're not a professional athlete and the only "victory" you can visualize is walking past the refrigerator without reaching inside for that tub of ice cream. The important thing is—whether your victory is on the soccer field or in the home gym—that you must visualize yourself enjoying physical movement.

It is key to imagine the *joy* of your workout, not just the work of your workout. This is especially important if you currently do not feel much joy about working out on your typical, average day. You need to get to a point where working out is less work and more fun; where the thought of suiting up and going to the gym or heading outside for a jog makes you smile instead of groan.

Start to mentally picture something that you enjoy doing, whatever it might be. Concentrate with all your mental powers on the smells, sounds, textures, appearance of the activity—the food, the person, the "whatever" that makes you feel good. Then begin to transfer those images to your workout.

This process is called transference. By merging the feelings you get from doing things you enjoy with working out, exercising *becomes* the thing you enjoy. In this way you can learn to look forward to your exercise the same way you look forward to a beer with dinner, a ball game, or time with your kids. It sounds impractical, but as we stated in the introduction to this section, it's been working for athletes for years. Now it's time to let it work for you.

This will be hardest at first. Even after you have an established pattern of enjoying your workouts, there will be days when you hate it and when you cannot imagine why you ever bothered going to the gym or lacing up your running shoes in the first place. Do not let your mind trick you into thinking you have failed. There are days when having a beer with dinner just gives you indigestion, when your team loses, and when your kids do not bring tears of joy to your eyes. Like you do with other things that are important to you, you remember that your team will play again and that your kids will be in better moods tomorrow. You think about that in order to get through today.

Visualization of results is important because it helps you discover what it is you truly want to gain from this program. When you can see something, you can more easily achieve it. This is particularly true when it comes to exercise; seeing the future tone of your body or the musculature you want to achieve is not only the ultimate motivator, it's the ultimate goal-producer.

EXERCISE:
Pre-Workout Visualization

Step 1: Go over in your mind what you plan on doing for the workout and the muscles you will be working.: biceps, calves, abdominals, etc.

Step 2: Picture one of those figures from your anatomy class. You know the kind, where you could see the muscles and sinews of the human body in cross section.

Step 3: Now take it one step further—see yourself lifting the repetitions and feeling the blood rushing to those muscles; you will feel the stretch, the burn, the extension, even the relaxing of the muscle. This isn't just to motivate you emotionally; by doing this, the mind will actually prepare your muscles for what is to come during the workout. This will help you overcome any hard exercises you may be trying at the gym.

Step 4: Imagine the results you want to achieve with this workout.

Step 5: Know that by doing this visualization exercise you have already started your workout. You are exercising out any doubt or confusion as to what you need to do. You are planning how effective your workout will be and what you want to achieve, and in so doing you are creating a self-fulfilling prophecy: by visualizing the muscles you want to exercise, the experience you want to have, the workout you hope to enjoy, your mind is preparing to help you achieve it.

EXERCISE:
Post-Workout Visualization

Just as we stretch before and after a workout, so too the visualization exercise doesn't end just because our workout is over.

Step 1: After you work out, you must first think about what you have just completed. Identify the parts that went well, and the parts that didn't.

Step 2: Think about all of the things that went right during your workout. As humans, we so often think about the negative first. In order to create more positive outcomes, from now on, begin looking at what's right. Reflect on all of the accomplishments you've achieved.

Step 3: Now recall the errors in your workout and figure out where you went wrong. Then spend time visualizing yourself doing the right thing. For example, if you realize that you did your E-Z Bar curls with too much momentum, visualize doing them without any momentum. Go through the visualization several times so that your brain becomes programmed to do the exercise correctly.

STEP # 3:
High Performance Meditation

Meditation usually refers to a state in which your body is consciously relaxed and the mind is allowed to become calm and focused. Although it often conjures up images of sitting in the "Lotus" position and staying still for hours, meditation doesn't necessarily have to be done that way. It is not necessary to be at home or in your "sacred" place, either. The wonderful thing about meditation is that it is possible to do virtually anywhere.

Most people claim that they cannot sit in silence and the thought of clearing their mind literally boggles, well, their *mind*. It certainly takes patience and some effort to allow the body and mind to "go quiet." With all we have to think about in our busy, hectic days—work commitments, appointments, kids' activities, dinner decisions, phone calls to make and return—clearing the mind can truly be a challenge.

Think of the last time you were truly relaxed. It might have been after seeing a particularly enjoyable movie, enjoying a great evening with friends, or going on a quick trip to some secluded hideaway where none of the daily pressures of life could penetrate.

What each of these relaxing episodes have in common is the absence of daily stressors, chores, and stimuli; you were removed from your day-to-day routine and the blur of life that accompanies it. As a result, you could relax and emerge from each experience refreshed, reinvigorated, and renewed. Now imagine feeling that way without paying for a movie ticket, party favors, or weekend getaway.

You can . . . through meditation.

When I go to the gym, I may feel anxiety, happiness, or anger. If I let these emotions control me, I would not be focused on my exercise. If I were to focus on my anger or anxiety, I could push too hard and seriously hurt myself. If I were to focus on just my happiness, I might become too relaxed and get nothing out of my workout.

High performance meditation is a tool that can help control our thoughts and feelings, so that they no longer control our minds and bodies. I've found that meditation improves every area of my life—there's that holistic connection again—so that all facets of my day benefit, not just my time at the gym. How and why do our feelings control our experiences and how can this positively help us to create great workouts?

If you looked at our bodies under the highest

magnification microscope, you would clearly see that we are all made of energy. All of our cells are made of molecules, which are made of atoms, which are made of subatomic particles such as electrons, which are energy.

All energy vibrates. Think of it like a tuning fork. When you tap a tuning fork it will vibrate with a certain pitched frequency. If there's a pile of other tuning forks lying around, only the tuning forks calibrated at the exact same frequency will respond, even if they are very far away from your original tuning fork.

This is precisely how our feelings help to create our actual reality. Just like the frequency of the tuning fork, we too are influenced by the vibrations that we emanate from our particular frequency. When we are feeling down and depressed, the vibrations associated with this particular frequency are low and will attract low frequencies. When you are feeling happy and joyful, the vibrations associated with this particular frequency will now be high and will naturally attract "happy" frequencies. This means you can consciously create states of happiness, at any time!

How? We simply need to assess our current moods periodically (every 15 minutes, if possible) to see what and how we're feeling. Here's an example: If you find that you are worrying about being too fat, guess what type of vibration and frequency this will be sending off and simultaneously magnetizing in? You guessed it, very low ones. When you stop worrying about being too fat and instead think about how healthy and happy you'll feel once you achieve fat loss, guess what? You have now set your vibration to a high setting, which will clearly attract the positive outcomes you so desire.

High performance meditation goes hand in hand with the visualization techniques you've just learned. High performance meditation calms and prepares your mind to be open to intense and enjoyable periods of visualization, much as visualization fosters a mental ease that translates well into meditation. Just like visualization, we practice before, during, and after our workouts.

Before your workout, you will meditate about how well you are doing and how well you will perform. Look for mental stumbling blocks and think about how you will overcome your fears of possible pain or failure to meet one of your goals. Face your fears and accept them; they are expected and they are not a big problem. By addressing your fears, by welcoming a positive workout experience, your mind is open to communing with the body in a more effective and joyful way.

During your workout is the most important time to use high performance meditation. In this instance you will meditate by listening to your body. When you feel tired or unable to continue, you say to yourself, "Okay, I knew this feeling would hit, just hang in there and it will pass. It's not so bad." That's it. Nothing mystical or New Age about it. Training yourself to constantly think this way during your exercise will help defend your body from negative thoughts.

After your workout, meditate on the workout you've just completed, focusing on the positives. For instance, suppose you had a difficult time one day because you were tired. The workout was so mediocre and the results so insignificant that you felt like giving up. Think about how good you feel for having stuck with it, what you can do better next time, and so on. After bad workouts I always tell my clients, "That's all right, that's okay. We'll live to fight another day . . " All I'm really doing with that phrase is vocalizing my internal meditation. It is important to do this exercise immediately after the workout for maximum results.

Here are some practical tips that will increase the effectiveness of your meditation sessions:

Tip 1: Before beginning a meditation session, you must be fully rested. Just as the body needs adequate rest for exercise and activity, the mind needs rest for concentration and focus. When you are tired, take a quick mental break and zone out for a few minutes. Also, try not to eat just before a session.

Tip 2: Set aside a specific time for practicing meditation. It will take only about 15 minutes a day to put the technique into action. But without a set time, procrastination can set in. By setting a specified time each day, such as right before sleep or upon rising in the morning, you will condition your mind to be ready and effective every day at the same time.

Tip 3: Be enthusiastic about your sessions. Don't think of them as hocus pocus or New Age hoo-haw; focus on the benefits and not the stigma. This works. Take pleasure in knowing that you are on your way to your best physique, even if you're not running or lifting weights.

Tip 4: When practicing meditation, you don't have to force it like exercise. In fact, you can't really force it. Take it easy and relax. We are not doing bodybuilding exercises, yet the results achieved will blow your mind. The more relaxed you are, the clearer your image will be, thus allowing for more powerful results.

For more information about meditation, visit www.digitalmeditation.com.

EXERCISE:
High Performance Meditation for Modifying Moods

Step 1: The first step in practicing meditation is to become entirely relaxed and calm. Try one of the relaxation techniques in Chapter 1.

Step 2: Stretch out comfortably on your favorite recliner or lie in your bed.

Step 3: Next, concentrate on one single point, either directly in front of you or above you, the ceiling for example.

Step 4: Begin by saying the following sentences either out loud or to yourself, consciously focusing on feeling the physical effects they produce on you. (Don't worry if you don't feel like memorizing these sentences right now; they are all included on the bonus CD for your convenience):

- "My mind is fully concentrating on my focal point and the harder I concentrate on this point the more my mind and body are relaxed." (Note: Take as much time as necessary to feel the intended effect of total relaxation. Take your time to honestly feel the relaxation set in.)

- "My eyes are getting more tired and my eyelids are get-ting heavier with every passing second." (Focus on your heavy eyelids as you fall deeper into your desired state).

- "I want to close my eyes, and I close my eyes."

- "I feel totally calm and relaxed. My body is getting heavier and heavier, sinking into my bed (or seat). I can feel myself so, so relaxed. My eyes are now completely closed and I am so, so relaxed, yet focused on my body." (Do not fall asleep, you are relaxed not sleepy.) "I will now begin to consciously relax my body." (Always begin with your feet, focusing first on your toes and moving body part by body part up toward your head.) Proceed as outlined below with the following suggestions.

- "I am concentrating all of my attention onto my feet, which are growing heavier and becoming so, so relaxed." (You may start to feel a tingling sensation as if very slight pins and needles were in your feet and toes.)

- "A very comfortable and warm feeling is vibrating throughout my entire body."

- "I will now focus on my legs, which are beginning to sink deeply into themselves." (Concentrate on this feeling but do not force it. This should be enjoyable, not work. When practiced regularly, you will automatically fall into the desired state quickly.)

- "My stomach is now beginning to feel very heavy, sinking deeper and deeper into itself." (Allow for relaxed and easy breathing to occur. As you progress and move on to each body part, simply allow that part to lazily relax while you concentrate on the amazing feelings of relaxing your body. What you are doing right now may very well change your life forever.)

- "My hands and fingers are growing heavier and heavier. They are totally relaxed."

- "My chest is now sinking deeper and deeper into itself. With each breath I fall deeper and deeper into relax-ation. I feel so, so calm and relaxed, I feel a warm vibration throughout my whole body."

- "My neck is growing heavy and feels so, so relaxed as I allow it to sink deeply into itself. My head is relaxing more and more. I feel no pressure, only the heaviness allowing my head to sink so deeply into itself. All of my thoughts are calming and relaxed. I feel as if I am floating in a dream."

- "In this mind state, every thought that I wish to focus on is so powerful, so very powerful that nothing can stop it from becoming reality, whatever the obstacles in my way." (Repeat this last sentence three times.)

Step 5: Now form a mental image of exactly what you want your mood to be when you begin your workout. Imagine the atmosphere of the gym, or your living room, if that's where you work out. See the weights and imagine hoisting them up. Now imagine how you want to feel; imagine the mood and frame of mind you want to be in during that time. Keep it in your mind's eye for about 10 to 15 minutes, without going over 15 minutes. If you start getting tired or tense, stop and rest for a few minutes before continuing.

Step 6: Think about your mood and reaction to the workout environment by concentrating all of your attention on it. Allow your mind and body to experience the emotion and attitude you want to have. The more you are absorbed by it, the stronger the effect, thereby creating greater success. The more the message is present in your mind during the session, the more easily your body and attitude will recreate that mood during the workout.

Step 7: Before beginning your next workout, recall the image you created during this exercise and allow your subconscious mind to recreate it in the present. If you are feeling depressed or tired, it may take longer for the meditation image to take effect.

STEP #4:
Conscious Creation

This book will be powerless if you don't believe in the results I promise and feel them as your very own. The only way to truly accomplish this all-important goal is to "expect great change." Conscious creation puts you in a place where your body is receptive to exercise and to change; it helps you focus on the task at hand so that you benefit more from what you're doing and do more of what you're there to do.

The best way for you to excel at what you do is to believe in yourself. Like I tell my clients, "Believe and you will achieve. Many exercisers have excuses not to work out. "I can't go jogging today because it's going to rain." "Thanksgiving is this Thursday and I know I'll overeat, so why work out this week at all?" "I've already done three sets, why do all five?" When this happens, you are consciously lying to yourself and you are not evolving in your physical fitness abilities.

One of the best ways to "excuse-proof" your workout is to make the "creation" of the workout program a part of your daily routine.

If you make working out part of your routine, then you will not spend time deciding whether or not you are going to work out. You just do it because you always do it. It is part of your life. You wouldn't think of not walking the dog, depositing your paycheck, making dinner, or taking a shower, would you? Likewise, when your workout becomes part of your daily routine you will hardly ever skip a workout again.

Another way to consciously create change in your abilities is to build on your success. Often people will begin to have doubts about their physical fitness. When a person begins working out and gradually evolves to lifting more and more weight, they will hit a wall where they can-

not go any farther. Although they have physically improved a great deal, mentally they feel like they lack energy. If you are tired, even the most tired you have ever been, remember that you will start feeling better when you reach your ultimate goal. Practicing the art of staying positive and remembering your successes. You will experience great changes, because you will have come up against and actually climbed over the wall to accomplish your goal.

It sounds easier than it is. I admit it. Achieving your ultimate body won't be easy, nor will achieving a proper balance between the body and mind when the two have been kept separate for so long. But you will get there; it will flow. The important thing to remember is that the tips and techniques I'm sharing with you in this section build upon one another, much like having stronger legs takes the strain off of your back or lifting weights in the gym translates into lifting your children easier in the morning. Setting goals helps you meditate, which helps you expect and consciously create great change.

Conscious creation is different from visualization and conviction exercises because instead of merely imagining results, you create the results. Use goal-setting to determine the path that you want to follow, then use visualization to develop your own beliefs in the ability of your body. For instance, use a pre-workout visualization to see yourself doing more repetitions than your last workout. Then, you must then consciously create the images by actually trying to do more repetitions.

EXERCISE:
Conscious Creation

Step 1: Imagine yourself reaching an attainable goal—for instance, doing additional repetitions of the lat pulldown—that you think is possible at the present time but have not actually tried yet.

Step 2: Next you must consciously create the goal by actively trying it. Use the imagery and constantly say to yourself, for example, "I have already done more repetitions." Think back to your imagery and trick your mind into believing that the imagery you conducted actually occurred.

Step 3: Then think to yourself that "since I did it before I can do it now."

Step 4: Do the additional repetitions.

STEP #5:
Guided Imagery

Guided imagery—using your imagination to cope with illness and stress more effectively—is rooted in the mind-body connection we have established and has been practiced throughout many cultures for hundreds, if not thousands, of years. The best way to describe the concept of guided imagery is to think of it as aromatherapy for the mind. You are trying to recapture good feelings that arose from various images or stimuli—sights, smells, sounds, experiences—in a "guided" way to help focus on healing or growth.

We have already discussed how your thoughts give rise to your emotions, which in turn affect your well-being. Visualizing positive images regarding your fitness regimen, workout, or jogging path can improve your performance by making a positive experience better and a negative experience more positive.

Let's use an image or scenario you might be able to relate to: you're having a bad workout and it's just not going well. The music in the gym stinks, you feel "off," your clothes are too tight or too loose, the lines for the machine are too long, you're just not "there." What guided imagery does is help you to recall images from a more positive workout and use them to recreate those feelings—kind of like the way thinking about a hot, juicy steak makes you crave a hot, juicy steak—so that you can turn a bad workout into a good one. The richer the details of your images are—colors, textures, smells, tastes, sounds—the more powerfully they work.

If the best thing that ever happened to you was the perfect song on the radio at the perfect time, then use the memories, visual and/or auditory, of that time to guide you further into a mindful, calm fitness practice. Whatever it is that brings lightness or joy to you is a memory worth bringing into every aspect of your life, even the practice of fitness.

Because guided imagery merges not only the mind and body, but also sight and sound, it can be very effective for those who have the most difficulty maintaining mindfulness while achieving their fitness goals. In November 2004, *World Disease Weekly* reported a study that suggested using guided imagery even briefly, measurably reduces psychological anxiety and the physical manifestations of anxiety in addition to improving memory.

This is not the only study that reported such effects. By using psychological techniques and mental processes that are proven to alleviate performance inhibiting anxiety, an athlete at whatever level of performance or competition can move him- or herself closer to the goals they have established.

EXERCISE:
Guided Imagery

Step 1: The next time your workout isn't going well, stop between exercises and take a break. Find a place where you can be quiet and by yourself for 5 to 10 minutes.

Step 2: Sit down and begin breathing in a calm and relaxed manner. Relax your muscles and close your eyes.

Step 3: Begin thinking about the last time you had a great workout. What were things like? How did you feel? What was your energy level? Recreate the image in your mind and allow your body to relive the vitality of the experience in the present tense. Allow the positive emotions and energy to sweep over you. Consciously notice the tension and frustration leaving your mind and body.

Step 4: Once you find yourself in a positive, energetic mood, return to your workout and go at it with a new sense of gusto.

STEP #6:
The Mind Over Muscle Activation Sheet

To create actual, constant, and long-lasting change in your life, you should work with these five techniques in the present tense. You create actual change now, not in the future. To that end I am including here something that works in concert with the *Mind Over Muscle* Journal I introduced in Chapter 1. I call it my *Mind Over Muscle* Activation Sheet and it is designed to help you do the following:

- List your goals;
- Get specific about short-term and long-term goals;
- Discuss your emotions in a beneficial manner;
- Set a concrete action plan for the coming day;
- Get the most of your self-actualization.

Like everything else we've discussed in this section, I've tried to make the Activation Sheet repeatable, useful, and habitual, so it can truly effect change in a way you've never experienced before.

Here's an analogy for you: Are you aware of the great difference between cardiovascular exercise and weight training? The effects of cardio exercise only last momentarily after the cardio session is over, while the effects of weight training last for hours after the actual training session. This has to do with muscle and the energy it creates and emits for long periods of time.

The *Mind Over Muscle* Activation Sheet acts just like the post-weight-training effects: The effects of the exercise continue long after the technique has been activated and engaged. What's even better is that it continues to work even when you stop paying attention. Visualization is short-lived. The worksheet I've designed can help you see the picture longer, and even "frame it" so that you can repeat the visualization over and over again.

In order to gain the most astounding results from the program, you must really make it a priority to fill out the *Mind Over Muscle* Activation Sheet every day—and to do it with ambition. Since it is specific and goal-oriented, I have designed the worksheet to be completed the day before a goal is to be achieved. This gives you time to "live with" your goal instead of just thinking one up on the spur of the moment.

The *Mind Over Muscle* Activation Sheet utilizes the power of human emotions. You must learn to fully feel and verbalize your emotions. I have even given you a space to outline your emotions about each goal, right there in black and white, so you don't forget. You have to decide what emotion you want to feel—self-confident, grateful, joyful, purposeful, worthy, energetic, etc.—and to feel this emotion in the present moment.

Emotions and feelings are not part of the typical exercise routine, I know. But it's important to identify the emotions you're targeting because by merely identifying them you are putting the cart in motion, so to speak; you will move much further and more quickly toward achieving your goals because you have created the perfect set of circumstances to help make your goals a reality.

It's not a goals sheet or action plan; it's an Activation Sheet. We're doing just that; we're "activating" your emotional investment in each and every workout, jog, or aerobics class. I'm very big on documenting, as you can probably tell, because I've found that my clients do better when they write better

It seems like a lot of work, I know. (Hey, it's not called a "worksheet" for nothing!) The thing is, it's important to give attention to your goals EVERY DAY. A workout without goals is like driving with no destination. It may be fun, but where does it get you?

Much like I suggest you begin getting comfortable with meditation techniques before we engage in the workouts they'll precede, I suggest that you begin creating concrete goals today and start filling in these worksheets throughout the rest of the book. Remember, goals start before workouts begin.

All of what I've tried to impart to you in this section has to do with visualizing: seeing what you want and attaining it by believing you can have it. That's it; it's that simple. Unfortunately, for many of us, it's the farthest thing from easy. We have been taught that exercise is physical and has nothing to do with the emotional. Now, thanks to science, we know better. Seeing the result of a workout is just as important as the workout; it's the feeling and belief that's associated with the goal that's most important and not just the goal itself.

Feelings are as important as muscle fiber; you must learn to feel what it's like to want the goal, reach the goal, and enjoy accomplishing what you've achieved. Only, we have to get you out of feeling it in that particular order! You want to feel as if you've accomplished the goal before you even set the goal. That, my dear readers, is what mindful preparation is all about.

And this is how you get there . . .

Worksheet # 1:

Sample Mind Over Muscle Activation Sheet

I've provided here my *Mind Over Muscle* Activation Sheet. On this page I've filled in an action plan based on several that my clients have created over the years. (While the real form has room for three goals—and you can always write more—I've only filled in two.)

You'll find a blank Activation Sheet in Appendix B that you can fill in as desired (using a pencil for multiple uses) or photocopy it and use it at will. Whichever way you choose, I do realize that many people do struggle with their emotions—resisting them, not always being able to properly identify them, and even being uncomfortable expressing them.

The wonderful thing about feeling your positive emotions as much as possible is that the emotions will help to transform into your solid reality. Enjoy the Activation Sheet, and may it bring you much goal-centered "activation" in the future:

Date: June 12, 2006
Time: 7:43 a.m.

Overall Assessment of this Day:

Overall, today was a good day. I feel better about how far I've come on the Mind Over Muscle Program and look forward to good things down the road as I get more comfortable with various tips and techniques like visualization and guided imagery. I wish I had more energy, but I know that will come with continued weight loss and getting used to exercising three times each week as opposed to two.

Assessment of the Day's Workout:

I think today's workout session went fairly well, although I had planned on staying longer than I did and doing more. Unfortunately, about three-quarters of the way to my goal I just ran out of energy. That's okay, though. I know that I did better today than I did the day before and, hopefully, will do better tomorrow, too.

Tomorrow's Goals:

Goal # 1: Tomorrow I intend to have more rest and eat closer to the time I work out (but not too close). I think the reason I ran out of energy today was because I ate too long before going to the gym and didn't hydrate myself properly.

Details of Goal # 1 (When, Why, How):

I had a lot on my mind and didn't sleep well last night, so felt sluggish when I woke up. To avoid repeating this tomorrow night I am going to turn off the TV sooner and meditate longer so that I will be more ready for sleep; sooner.

Emotion You Connect with Goal # 1:

I am encouraged that by doing something as simple as turning off the boob tube half an hour earlier I can affect how I feel in the morning. I am also looking forward to mastering my art of meditation, which I have been slacking on for the last week or so. I know the techniques—I have that part of the book dog-eared—but I have been focusing on the physical instead of the mental for too long. Now I am eager to have a healthier mix of mind AND body!!!

Goal # 2:

In addition to having more rest and eating later in the afternoon, I plan on hydrating myself better so that I don't feel too high or low during my workout, but instead have a steadier flow of energy.

Details of Goal # 2 (When, Why, How):

To accomplish this goal I will drink water on the way to the gym and have a bottle of water with me while I work out. I can either buy a bottle of water on the way to the gym and replenish it when I get there or buy a sports bottle at the drug store and replenish it before I go to the gym and once I get there.

Emotion You Connect with Goal # 2:

I am excited that by taking such a simple step as hydrating myself I can actually increase my stamina during a workout and remain focused longer. I am also disappointed that I didn't think of it sooner!

Chapter 3:

Mindful Nutrition

Proper Fueling for a Perfect Body—

The What, the When & the Why's

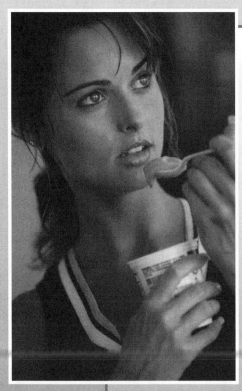

"Eating blindly" can be at the root of many of our health, weight, and even fitness dilemmas—without us even realizing it. Mindful nutrition, then, is the polar opposite of eating blindly; it is paying attention to what we put in our mouths—being mindful about what we eat—with the knowledge that what we consume affects the quality of our performance, body, mind, and soul.

Many books refer to food as the fuel for a good workout; I contend that proper nutrition is also the key that starts the ignition, the gears that allow you to move, and the very frame that supports the engine. Without the right nutrients in the correct quantities, the body will not be able to operate at peak performance levels and neither will the mind.

In this book, I present you with a sensible and realistic program that will result in optimal mental clarity, tons of energy, new muscle, and best of all, a reduction in body fat! Specifically in this section, we'll be talking about the following keys to healthy eating:

1. Mood Foods
2. Calorie Allocation
3. The 40/40/20 Rule
4. The Perfect Meal Plan

Speaking of body fat, this is a good place to mention that if your goal is less body fat, concentrate on just that, rather than on losing weight. The problem with focusing on weight loss is that weight includes lean muscle tissue, bone density, water, skin, organs and everything else that make up your entire body. To burn excess body fat, you simply need to burn off more calories than you consume. It's that easy!

If you've eaten 2,000 calories, than you will need to burn off those calories by the end of that day. Now, please understand, you won't be able to—nor should you attempt to—burn all of those calories in one cardio session. The overall calories burned by the end of the day are all a result of every moment of the day past. In other words, from the moment you awake to the moment you go to bed and even beyond, you are burning calories.

"So," you might ask, "why should I eat so many calories if I'm only trying to burn those calories off anyway? Why don't I just not eat very much at all?" Great question! The answer is simple: Your body needs calories in order to create energy, which allows you to function and train. The more quality fuel you put into your body, the more quality output you will ultimately receive.

Having said that, let's start covering some nutrition basics so that you can be *mindful* of what you put in your mouth, and not just *full*. In order to run a human body; you need six major nutrients. They are carbohydrates, protein, vitamins, minerals, water, and fat. Carbohydrates are our main source of food energy. Those flourish in grains, legumes, fruits, vegetables, and starches. Protein plays an important role in your growth and the repair of your body tissues and abounds in grains, legumes,

meat, dairy, and green vegetables. Vitamins are compounds that help regulate chemical reactions in the body. Minerals are important for the normal functioning of the body. Vitamins and minerals are used to metabolize all these nutrients and are found in green and yellow vegetables. Water is essential for a healthy body, makes up about 2/3 of your body weight, and is freely available. Fat is an important form of concentrated fuel for your body that should be consumed in limited quantities.

Foods contain combinations of nutrients. Contrary to what the lobbyists for the fruit or milk groups might tell you, no single food can supply all nutrients in the amounts you need. For example, oranges provide vitamin C but no vitamin B12; cheese provides vitamin B12 but no vitamin C. To make sure you get all of the nutrients and other substances needed for optimum health, you have to choose the recommended number of daily servings from each of the five major food groups displayed in the food guide pyramid.

Meat, Poultry, Fish, Dry Beans, Eggs & Nuts Group
2-3 Servings

Milk, Yogurt & Cheese Group
2-3 Servings

Fruit Group
2-4 Servings

Vegetable Group
3-5 Servings

Bread, Cereal, Rice & Pasta Group
6-11 Servings

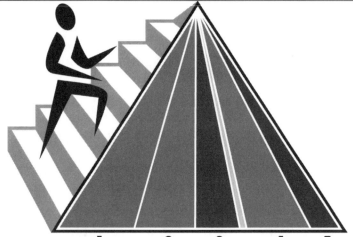

MyPyramid.gov
STEPS TO A HEALTHIER YOU

1) Grain Group: Make half your grains whole
- Eat at least 3 oz. of whole-grain cereals, breads, crackers, rice, or pasta every day
- 1 oz. is about 1 slice of bread, about 1 cup of breakfast cereal, or 1/2 cup of cooked rice, cereal, or pasta

2) Vegetable Group: Vary your veggies
- Eat more dark green veggies like broccoli, spinach, and other dark leafy greens
- Eat more orange vegetables like carrots and sweet potatoes
- Eat more dry beans and peas like pinto beans, kidney beans, and lentils

3) Fruit Group: Focus on fruits
- Eat a variety of fruit
- Choose fresh, frozen, canned, or dried fruit
- Go easy on fruit juices

4) Milk Group: Get your calcium-rich foods
- Go low-fat or fat-free when you choose milk, yogurt, and other milk products
- If you don't or can't consume milk, choose lactosefree products or other calcium sources such as fortified foods and beverages

5) Meat & Beans Group: Go lean with protein
- Choose low-fat or lean meats and poultry
- Bake it, broil it, or grill it
- Vary your protein routine — choose more fish, beans, peas, nuts, and seeds

Find your balance between food and physical activity
- Be sure to stay within your daily calorie needs.
- Be physically active for at least 30 minutes most days of the week.
- About 60 minutes a day may be needed to prevent weight gain.
- For sustaining weight loss, at least 60 to 90 minutes a day may be required.
- Children and teenagers should be physically active for 60 minutes every day, or most days.

Know the limits on fats, sugars, and salt (sodium)
- Make most of your fat sources from fish, nuts, and vegetable oils.
- Limit solid fats like butter, stick margarine, shortening, and lard, as well as foods that contain these.
- Check the Nutrition Facts label to keep saturated fats, trans fats, and sodium low.
- Choose food and beverages low in added sugars. Added sugars contribute calories with few, if any, nutrients.

Mood Foods

If you don't think foods affect your mood, try sitting still after eating a bar of chocolate or taking a walk around the block after dining on a heaping helping of pasta! Yes, there are such things as mood foods.

Remember that our moods are chemical; our emotions, our thoughts, our feelings, our motivations, our desires are all electrical impulses sent by our brains based on, and fed by, chemicals we have ingested at one time or another. When you eat, you should picture yourself in a laboratory, white lab coat and all, carefully preparing for a chemical reaction that will eventually go on inside your body once you eat.

In our modern, fast-paced world it is very, very easy to go an entire day without ingesting a single piece of fresh, natural, REAL food. From the drive-thru window on the way to work or the breakfast bar during rush hour traffic to the vending machine bags that make up our lunch to the microwave or boxed dinners we wolf down in front of the TV—and all the pre-packaged snacks in between—we're creating in our bodies a chemical cocktail that can't help but affect our moods.

We're happy on Monday, we reach for a certain type of food to enhance, feed, or prolong that happiness. We're sad on Wednesday so we reach for another type of food to make us feel better. Some moods make us reach for more food; some moods make us reach for less. Oftentimes the food we eat doesn't just enhance our mood, but actually creates it! By studying what we eat when we're emotional, we can not only pinpoint our emotional eating but likewise identify the foods that make us emotional in the first place.

Which Foods Produce Bad Moods?

For instance, eating an increased amount of red meats, cheeses, and sweets can often be an indicator of something wrong in your life, such as tension or stress. Not surprisingly, all of these items are high in fat. Participants in one study who had previously specified that food helps them "to cope" and "cheers them up" were significantly more likely to eat sweet food and cheese (a high-fat food) during the so-called "high-stress weeks." Finally, men were likely to eat more red meat during high-stress weeks, while women were not. (*Calm Energy: How People Regulate Mood with Food and Exercise*, 2003)

Why? The human body is still drawn to its prehistoric roots. The body senses danger and stress and therefore believes it needs to increase fat intake in order to survive. Of course, in the old days, stress meant physical danger or potential starvation; today it means an overbearing boss, looming deadlines, or a weekend with the in-laws! If you find yourself eating more red meats, cheeses, and sweets, then ask yourself what is stressing you out.

How do these foods contribute to our bad moods? They contain more than their fair share of these problematic ingredients:

Refined and Added Sugars: Refined and added sugars are "linked to poor concentration, mood swings, hyperactivity, aggression, nightmares, cravings, panic attacks, asthma, allergies, tiredness and anxiety." ("Body Talk: Ultimate Family Food") Sugar is one of the most harmful substances for your body because of the extremes it causes inside the delicate internal balance that regulates your body. Refined and added sugars are fast-acting carbs that can create a surge of energy and an upbeat mood followed by a big slump.

Stimulants: Stimulants like caffeine (found in sweets and soft drinks) have no place in your diet. Can you afford to start a program of physical activity and be continually tired? Stimulants make you "feel temporarily more alert and energetic, but leave you depressed and with a lack of energy once the drug wears off." ("Body Talk: Ultimate Family Food")

Hydrogenated Fats: Hydrogenated fats, found in most processed foods, cause you to be sluggish and your reaction time and motivation is cut short by interfering with the ability of your nerves to signal to your brain.

Refined Carbs: Refined carbs, like white flour or white rice, are stripped of fiber, vitamins, minerals, and other nutrients. These foods are problematic not because of what they contain but because of all of the nutrition they *lack*.

An aside about high-protein, low-carb diets: Carb consumption is associated with sunnier moods, so people following a high-protein, low-carb diet over a long period of time may be at an increased risk of depression. ("Body Talk: Happy Meals")

If you are more depressed, then guess what will happen to you? That's right: you will begin to eat more red meats, cheeses, and sweets. As a result of your carb-free diet, you will gain more weight and fat, and lack energy and remain depressed. Suddenly, the low-carb diet does not seem so appealing, does it?

Which Foods Produce Good Moods?

So, now that you're aware, you can stop yourself from automatically reaching for that chocolate bar to comfort you in a time of stress. Even better, you can substitute foods that can help you feel better.

Omega-3 Fats: Scientists have found that eating oily fish, which contain omega-3 fats, may prevent depression, promote learning, and improve memory. ("Body Talk: Feeling Grumpy? . . .") Good sources of this type of fat include salmon, sardines, mackerel, tuna, walnuts, flaxseed, and omega-3 enriched eggs—all of which are also high in protein. This makes sense: a protein-rich diet can help to "even out" moods by maintaining blood sugar levels and increasing your alertness and energy.

Selenium: A low intake of selenium has been found in people with depression. Selenium is also found in omega-3 enriched eggs and in Brazil nuts, cereals, meat, fish, and cheese.

B Vitamins: The B vitamins, especially folic acid and thiamin, contribute to a better mood and help boost your immune system so that you recover more quickly from strenuous workouts. Folic acid is found in liver and dark green, leafy vegetables. Thiamin will help stave off depression and is found in whole grain foods, fortified breakfast cereals, nuts, meat (particularly pork), peas, and orange juice. An easy way to include more thiamin in your diet is to simply switch from white rice, bread, and pasta to brown or whole-grain items. In addition, the carbs in these foods give you energy and contribute to a sunnier disposition.

Magnesium: Magnesium, a mineral that helps your mind and body relax, will reduce your stress as a result. Spinach and sunflower seeds are good sources of magnesium.

Tryptophan: Similarly, tryptophan, found in bananas and turkey, helps calm and relax you for a good night's sleep. Bananas, together with B-vitamin-rich oats, are my favorite remedy for insomnia.

You may have noticed that most of the "bad mood foods" are also "unhealthy foods"—that is, they also contribute to overweight and obesity, heart disease, cancer, and many other diseases—whereas the "good mood foods" are "good for you"—that is, they are full of wholesome nutrition and can help you lose weight and fend off many diseases. Since, as we've been learning, the health of our mind and our body is inextricably linked, this should be no surprise.

Calorie Allocation

When it comes to the reasons why you decided to plunk down your money for this book, I would like to think that the mind-muscle connection was enough of a reason but I suspect a lot of the rationale had to do with FAT. What is it, how do you get rid of it and, more importantly, how do you keep it off? In this section, we answer all three of those questions and many more.

The good news is that the secret of fat loss is actually pretty simple:

1. Create a slight caloric deficit. In other words, you need to eat slightly fewer calories than what you burn every day. For most men this is approximately 1,500 to 2,000 calories and for most women this is approximately 1,200 to 1,500.
2. Follow the 40/40/20 Rule. Eat roughly 40% carbohydrates, 40% proteins, and 20% fats.
3. Eat six small meals throughout the day. This gives you more stable energy levels, fewer cravings, and increased metabolism. You will be feeding your mind and your body every two to three hours; now that's truly mindful nutrition.

MOOD FOODS CHART

Good Mood Foods	Bad Mood Foods
Bananas *Tryptophan*	**RealFruit Juices (Diluted)** *B-vitamins, vitamin C*
Caffeinated Drinks, Energy Drinks *caffeine, refined sugar*	**Rye Bread** *Whole grain flour*
Chocolate *Caffeine, fat, refined sugar*	**Salmon and Other Fish** *Omega-3 fats, protein, selenium*
Cooking Oil *hydrogenated fats*	**Skim Milk** *Protein, calcium*
Fast Food *refined carbs, refined sugar, hydrogenated fats*	**Spinach** *Magnesium, folic acid*
Flaxseed *Omega-3 fats, protein*	**Steak and Other Red Meat** *fats*
Hot Dogs and Sandwich Meats *hydrogenated fats, preservatives*	**Sunflower Seeds** *Magnesium, protein*
Ice Cream *hydrogenated fats*	**Unsalted Peanuts** *Omega-3 fats, protein*
Multi-Grain Cereal *Whole grains, B-vitamins*	**Walnuts** *Omega-3 fats, protein*
Oranges *B-vitamins, vitamin C*	**White Bread, Croissants, White Rolls** *refined carbs*
Pastries and Cakes *refined carbs, refined sugar, hydrogenated fats*	**White Pasta** *refined carbs*
Pizza *refined sugar, hydrogenated fats*	**White Rice** *refined carbs*
	Whole Wheat Bread *Whole grain flour*
	Yogurt (Fat and Sugar Free) *Protein, calcium*
	Real

EXERCISE:
DAILY CALORIC INTAKE

Step 1: Before you start cutting or adding calories to your eating plan, first you need to address what it is you are trying to achieve. In other words, are you trying to lose weight or, more correctly, *lose body fat?* Are you trying to gain some lean muscle tissue? Are you just trying to maintain your current weight? Depending on your answers, your caloric intake will vary. Note that the following figures are not set in stone and your daily caloric intake should be slightly adjusted based on your individual needs and goals.

Step 2: For men, because you are more muscular, you'll need a minimum of about 1,500 to 2,000 calories per day in caloric intake. Women, you should aim for at least a 1,200 to 1,500 calorie diet. Regardless of sex, you should never reduce you daily calorie intake to less than 1,200 calories without medical or dietician supervision.

Step 3: If you want to lose weight, remove 500 calories per day. If you're after muscle gain, add 500 calories. Try this for 1 to 2 weeks and record your weight before and after. Be careful not to lose too much too quickly. There has been evidence that losing more than 0.5 to 1.0 pounds per week may severely burn muscle and dramatically decrease metabolism.

Step 4: To accurately track your body fat to lean muscle ratio, take a body fat test. This way you can see exactly where you stand with your ratio. There are plenty of great body fat testing procedures. One of the most accurate and least expensive tools is the Body Fat Analyzer HBF-306 from Omron (priced between $39.00 and $56.00). Whether you are male or female, try to maintain your lean muscle tissue. Muscle constantly burns calories, so you should strive never to lose muscle mass.

Step 5: Eat according to the activity you plan to be doing in the next three hours. Ideally, you'll want to consume about six small meals per day, every three hours, starting with breakfast. The exception to the rule is if you train shortly after you wake up; then you can always eat anything before you exercise, since you can take advantage of a fat-burning metabolism.

See the chart on the next page for an example of how you should allocate your daily caloric intake according to your activity level. If cravings besiege you in the evenings, as they do many of us, you can eat a high protein snack (i.e. low-fat yogurt or cottage cheese) at around 10:00 p.m. or about one hour before bedtime.

The 40/40/20 Rule

In following the 40/40/20 rule, it's important not only to eat carbohydrates, proteins, and fats in the right proportions but to eat the right type of each nutrient.

Carbohydrates:
Fuel for the Mind and the Muscle

Carbohydrates are the mind and body's primary source of energy. Carbohydrates are classified as complex or simple. The complex carbohydrates are further divided into starches like brown rice, sweet potatoes, oatmeal, and whole grain breads, and fibrous carbohydrates like green beans, broccoli, lettuce, tomatoes, and so on. In general, simple carbohydrates are released more quickly into the bloodstream. If they are not burned immediately through some sort of physical activity, they have a tendency to be stored as body fat. Complex carbohydrates, on the other hand, are usually released more slowly and thus offer more sustained energy levels.

The glycemic index measures more exactly which carbs are released at what rates. For optimal fat loss we want to stick with the lower to medium glycemic index carbohydrates throughout the day—those which are released more slowly. You can have higher glycemic index carbs—those which are released more quickly—immediately after a workout as research shows that at that time, the body needs carbohydrates to replenish those burned and to re-start the muscle building process. The list below will give you a good idea of which carbohydrates are low glycemic and which ones are high, as well as the best times to eat them.

Lower to Medium Glycemic
Complex Starchy Carbohydrates

Because of their slow-burning potential, these types of starchy carbohydrates are best eaten throughout the day.

- Old-fashioned oatmeal
- Barley
- Brown rice
- Cream of wheat
- Sweet potatoes
- Spaghetti
- White rice
- Pumpernickel bread
- Chickpeas

Higher Glycemic Complex
Starchy Carbohydrates

These types of carbohydrates are released into the body more quickly than those on the previous list. As a result, they are best eaten after a workout, when the body needs carbohydrates desperately in order to replenish those burned and to re-start the muscle building process.

- Cream of rice
- Grits
- Most breads
- Instant rice

CALORIE ALLOCATION CHART

(You should be eating at
6, 9, 12, 3, 6, & 8:30)

PERIOD 1: (6am – 9am)
Light activity (i.e. getting
ready to start your day)
MEN: 200 calories   WOMEN: 150 calories

PERIOD 2: (9am – 12pm)
Light/moderate activity
(i.e. doing daily chores)
MEN: 300 calories   WOMEN: 250 calories

PERIOD 3: (12pm – 3pm)
Moderate activity (i.e. walking around)
MEN: 300 calories   WOMEN: 200 calories
*One and a half hours before your
workout, eat a piece of fruit or a
food source containing fructose
for sustained energy.

PERIOD 4: (3pm – 6pm)
Physical training session
(i.e. weight training)
MEN: 600 calories   WOMEN: 500 calories

PERIOD 5: (6pm – 9pm)
Moderate activity (i.e. shopping)
MEN: 200 calories   WOMEN: 100 calories

PERIOD 6: (8:30pm)
1 hour post workout meal
MEN: 200 calories   WOMEN: 150 calories
*One hour after your workout,
drink a protein/carbohydrate
shake for replenishment :

PERIOD 7: (9pm – 11pm)
Sedentary activity (i.e. sleep)
MEN: 200 calories   WOMEN: 150 calories

- Instant mashed potatoes
- Rice cakes

Lower Glycemic Complex Fibrous Carbohydrates

I recommend that you eat these throughout the day; there are no higher glycemic fibrous carbs.

- Green Beans
- Broccoli
- Lettuce
- Cauliflower
- Tomato
- Spinach
- Turnip Greens
- Zucchini
- Asparagus
- Artichokes
- Okra
- Cabbage
- Heart of Palm
- Cucumbers
- Celery
- Dill Pickles
- Radishes
- Broccoli
- Brussels Sprouts
- Eggplant
- Onions
- Cauliflower
- Bell Peppers
- Green Peas
- Squash

Lower to Medium Glycemic Simple Carbohydrates

Limit to two servings per day, in breakfast and after a workout. Even though they are lower glycemic, simple carbs *do* tend to get stored as body fat.

- Grapefruit
- Apples, dried
- Prunes
- Apples, raw
- Pears
- Plums
- Strawberries
- Oranges
- Grapes

High Glycemic Simple Carbohydrates

Limit to *after* a workout only:

- Bananas
- Kiwi
- Apricots Dried or Fresh
- Papaya
- Pineapple
- Figs
- Raisins
- Cantaloupe
- Watermelon

Proteins: Mind Over Muscle Food

Proteins provide the body with the amino acids it needs for tissue repair and cellular growth. All tissues in the body have some protein in them, including hair, skin, and finger- and toenails. Muscles also are made up from protein. Proteins also increase the metabolism by 20% when ingested and help time-release the metabolism of carbs. In other words, when one combines proteins and carbohydrates in the same meal, proteins serve to bring down the glycemic index of the carbohydrates due to the fact that proteins are very complex molecules that require plenty of digestion.

Everybody who is doing a weight training program, such as the one presented in this book, should consume at least 1 gram of protein per pound of body weight. While more protein can be ingested, it is not necessary to go above 1.5 times your bodyweight in grams of protein.

Good examples of protein are lean sources such as:

- Egg whites
- Chicken breast (skinless)
- Turkey breast (skinless)
- 95% lean red meats
- Tuna
- Wild Alaskan salmon

On the other hand, proteins to stay away from include:

- High fat red meats
- Deli meats as they are high in sodium and sometimes are even sweetened with sugars!
- Any processed meats like hot dogs, bologna, sausages, bacon, ham, etc.

Fats: Brain and Hormone Food

Contrary to what most people think, *eating* fat does not necessarily make you fat. Again, the culprit for weight gain is taking in more calories than what you burn on a consistent basis. Fat, believe it or not, is of utmost importance to our nutrition program. Eliminate all fats from your diet and your brain will not be able to operate efficiently and your hormonal production will go down as well. Why does that matter? Hormones involved in the muscle-building and fat-burning process, like testosterone, require good fats in order to be manufactured.

Saturated Fats

Saturated fats are associated with heart disease and high cholesterol levels. They are found to a large extent in products of animal origin. However, some vegetable fats are altered in a way that increases the amount of saturated fats by a chemical process known as hydrogenation.

Stay away from:
- hydrogenated vegetable oils
- coconut oil
- palm oil
- palm kernel oil
- non-dairy creamers

Polyunsaturated Fats

These fats, unlike their saturated counterparts, do not ad-versely affect cholesterol levels and also remain liquid at room temperature. They are an essential element of the diet as they include a special family of essential fatty acids called omega 3 and omega 6 fatty acids. These fats are found in:
- safflower
- corn
- sunflower
- soybean oil
- flaxseed oil
- fish oils

Monounsaturated Fats

These fats actually lower bad cholesterol and may assist in reducing heart disease as well. They also provide essential fatty acids for healthy skin and the development of body cells, and also offer antioxidant properties. Good sources include:
- flaxseed
- fish oil
- olive oil

The Perfect Meal Plan

Eating six meals in a day won't be easy at first, but once you feel the effects of a faster metabolism and fewer blood sugar issues, I'm sure you'll agree that it's an avenue worth pursuing. To help your body optimize your food intake and energy reserves, your food choice and number of calories should be determined according to what

WATER:
THE KEY TO ULTIMATE VITALITY

In addition to the carbs, proteins, and fats you've calculated for yourself under the 40/40/20 Rule, you need to drink plenty of water. Water functions as a solvent for all the biochemical reactions taking place in the body; it also acts as a coolant, a means for release of toxins, and as a lubricant. The amount of water you'll need to consume each day varies for every single person on the planet. As a general rule, you should plan on drinking at least 0.66 times your body weight in ounces of water per day. Of course, variables such as time of year, physical activity, or lack thereof, all affect the body's need for water. In these cases, feel free to drink more in hot conditions or when exercising.

kind of activity you will be performing in the three hours following the time you eat. In other words, when you eat, you are, in fact, eating for a period of time about three hours ahead.

The importance of thinking ahead to form a solid eating plan that works for your lifestyle cannot be overstated. For example, a balanced breakfast can improve your mind, your energy level, your mood and help promote weight control. If you skip breakfast, you lower your stamina, endurance, and ability to concentrate, and you put yourself at risk for overeating and making less healthful choices later in the day. Eating breakfast also boosts metabolism and therefore you will burn calories more efficiently throughout the day.

Thinking ahead may sound complicated at first but it's no different than, say, watching the Weather Channel to determine what to pack for your vacation.

Basically, all you need to do is plan to have real food at breakfast, lunch, and dinner.

In between, have snacks, which can be in the form of either real food or protein shakes, bringing you up to your six full meals for the day. See the boxes for sample meal plan for men and women.

Cheat Day: Make Sunday Your "Funday"

For one meal each Sunday (or whatever day of the week you choose—so long as it's just one day), I want you to cheat on your diet. That's right, I insist that you go to your favorite restaurant and eat to your heart's desire. Just remember, it's one meal . . . one appetizer, one entrée and one dessert. (Of course, you should only reward yourself in this way if you've stayed on track for the rest of the week.)

Deviate from this by eating too much and you certainly risk taking a step backward, but stick to it and you won't harm your diet one bit. In fact, you will most likely increase your chance of staying on it. Here's why: having one cheat-meal a week can actually be most beneficial because it confuses your body and increases your metabolism. By cheating, you prevent your body from adjusting or adapting to the diet. It also removes the psychological fear associated with feeling like you'll never eat "bad" foods again.

Having said that, some people find it extremely difficult to revert back to "good" foods once they indulge for even this one meal. Despite their best intentions, they fall into a non-stop eating binge. Do not feel bad if you fall into this category. It is very natural to crave foods that are not so good for us. If you do fall into this category, please avoid this once a week cheat meal until you have reached a confident level of empowerment.

LIQUIDS, POWDERS AND SUPPLEMENTS

Supplements, powders, and shakes can help build stronger, leaner bodies. Powdered supplements provide a convenient way to add protein to your diet, particularly if you are constantly on the go.

Meal Replacement Powders typically contain carbohydrates, some good fats, and some vitamins and minerals as well. Go to your local Vitamin Shoppe to find a quality meal replacement.

Protein Powders are just straight protein with very few carbs (2 to 3 per scoop). For the most part, no vitamins and minerals are added.

Supplements

Since many foods these days are so processed, it is virtually impossible to get all of the vitamins and minerals one needs from food alone. Therefore, I recommend a good "one-a-day" type of multiple vitamin and mineral formula at breakfast time, 3 grams of vitamin C a day split between breakfast, lunch and dinner, 200 mcg of chromium picolinate (if not included with your vitamin/mineral pack) with breakfast, and 100 mg of alpha lipoic acid with breakfast, lunch and dinner.

NUTRITIONAL PLAN FOR MEN

Breakfast:
6:00 AM
- Choose a serving of low to medium glycemic index starchy carbs
- Choose a serving of low to medium glycemic index simple carbs
- Choose a serving of lean proteins

Snack #1:
10:00 AM
- Choose a serving of low to medium glycemic index starchy carbs
- Choose a serving of lean proteins
- Add a tablespoon of flaxseed oil

Lunch:
12:00 PM
- Choose a serving of low to medium glycemic index starchy carbs
- Choose a serving of fibrous carbs
- Choose a serving of lean proteins

Snack #2:
3:00 PM
- Choose a serving of low to medium glycemic index starchy carbs
- Choose a serving of lean proteins

Dinner:
6:00 PM
- Choose a serving of low to medium glycemic index starchy carbs
- Choose a serving of fibrous carbs
- Choose a serving of lean proteins
- Add a tablespoon of canned extra virgin olive oil to vegetables

Snack #3:
9:30 PM
- Choose a serving of low to medium glycemic index starchy carbs
- Choose a serving of low to medium glycemic index simple carbs
- Choose a serving of lean proteins

NOTE: This plan assumes a late evening workout from 8-9PM

*A serving of carbs is approximately 1 cup; a serving of protein, approximately 6 ounces.

NUTRITIONAL PLAN FOR WOMEN

Breakfast:
6:00 AM
Choose half a serving of low to medium glycemic index starchy carbs
Choose half a serving of low to medium glycemic index simple carbs
Choose half a serving of lean proteins

Snack #1:
10:00 AM
Choose half a serving of low to medium glycemic index starchy carbs
Choose half a serving of lean proteins
Add a tablespoon of flaxseed oil

Lunch:
12:00 PM
Choose half a serving of low to medium glycemic index starchy carbs
Choose half a serving of fibrous carbs
Choose half a serving of lean proteins

Snack #2:
3:00 PM
Choose half a serving of low to medium glycemic index starchy carbs
Choose half a serving of lean proteins

Dinner:
6:00 PM
Choose half a serving of low to medium glycemic index starchy carbs
Choose half a serving of fibrous carbs
Choose half a serving of lean proteins
Add a tablespoon of Canned Extra Virgin Olive Oil to vegetables

Snack #3:
9:30 PM
Choose half a serving of higher glycemic index starchy carbs
Choose half a serving of higher glycemic index simple carbs
Choose half a serving of lean proteins

NOTE: This plan assumes a late evening workout from 8-9PM

*A serving of carbs is approximately 1 cup; a serving of protein, approximately 6 ounces.

PRE- AND POST-WORKOUT MEALS

Knowing what to eat before and after a workout, can be just as important as the workout itself. Just like some foods put you in a better mood and others bring you down, so too must pre- and post-workout meals be chosen carefully so as to get the most out of your physical efforts.

For a pre-workout meal it is good to include carbohydrates that are healthy and not filled with fats or sugar. Cereals, whole wheat breads, and even oatmeal are excellent sources of carbohydrates that are good for you and can help fill you with energy. A single cup of coffee can also provide some quick energy and get your blood pumping. Peanut butter is a good source of protein, which you will need to build the muscles that you are about to start working out in your training program. As always, you will want to sip water before, during, and after your workout in order to stay hydrated. Stay away from sport drinks because these have a lot of sugar and can do more harm than good.

Post-workout meals are important because your body is in a vulnerable position after expending all that energy. Drink plenty of water to help re-hydrate your body. Eat green leafy vegetables and lean items that contain protein, like chicken, fish or lean red meats. A turkey sandwich after working out will help you calm down and help you relax so your body can better repair itself and further build itself up. Turkey contains tryptophan, which causes the body to relax. Drink a well-formulated carbohydrate/protein shake approximately one hour after a training session, when your body will absorb more of its nutrients.

Chapter 4:

Mindful Exercise

Get Into the Zone-Tone

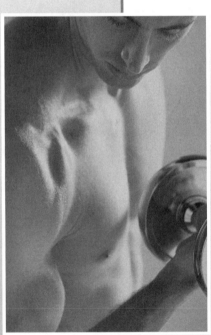

So far we've talked a lot about the mind and its crucial role in health and fitness. But our goal is to get you started on an exercise program that takes you directly to your fitness goals. The actual exercises and program begin in Part Two, but in this chapter we bring the mental training we've been talking about together with the exercises we're going to talk about. Think of it this way: At the crossroads of Parts One and Two of this book, the theory and practice of the mind-body connection meet at last!

I call that intersection "Mindful Exercise."

Mindful Exercise is about paying attention to the way you do your exercise. This chapter equips you with several tools to help you do just that. We're going to start with the "Zone-Tone" and "Two-Step Rep" techniques, which are essential to the program coming up in Part Three. That's followed by several techniques you can use to add variety, fun, and challenge to your program.

Keep in mind that these techniques can apply to many facets of everyday life. Experiment with the Two-Step Rep or use the Zone-Tone principles when you've got a deadline at work, or the Full Body Tension technique for lifting heavy things in your garage. Remember that the *Mind Over Muscle* philosophy is all about creating the best body you can achieve for living the best life you can live. So take and learn these techniques in your exercise program, then experiment with them in other parts of your life.

EXERCISE:
Getting into the Zone-Tone

The Zone-Tone is the art of mentally zoning in and pre-isolating specific muscles just before an exercise is to be executed while at the same time maintaining that zone throughout the execution of the movement. This means knowing precisely what muscles you are targeting before you start the exercise and moving the muscle from its fully extended position to its fully contracted position (full range of motion), while consciously focusing on feeling the muscles (and only the intended muscles) contract and extend throughout the entire movement.

When you effectively communicate with a specific muscle and prepare it for the upcoming set (work load), you have successfully engaged the mind-to-muscle connection. By keeping this connection active throughout the duration of the exercise, just that one set can produce the results of five sets! You're no longer splitting your time between mind to muscle and back again. Now you're engaging in the mind-body connection so that every rep is effective, every set is a great set.

The Zone-Tone method is made up of two simple steps:

Step 1: Focus and zone in on the individual muscle(s) you intend to train before you begin the exercise: Tense and contract (flex) the muscle to be trained as hard as comfortably possible before you even start to execute the exercise. This way you will be sending a message to that muscle, preparing it by completely isolating it even before the exercise begins. By doing so you have successfully created a mind-to-muscle connection.

Step 2: Maintain your mind-to-muscle connection during the execution of the exercise: Throughout the execution of the exercise, deliberately feel the muscle elongate (stretch) and contract (flex), as you move along from point A to point B (the full range of movement for a particular exercise).

What I really want you to do while you are performing the exercise is to contract (flex) the muscle as hard as you can in the same way that you did in step one, but with the exception that now you'll have a weight in your hand.

EXERCISE:
The Two-Step Rep

This technique regulates the tempo at which you move the weight through the range of motion in an exercise. I've chosen the Two-Step Rep technique for this program because it slows you down so that you can fully engage your mind in the process of each repetition. As you focus on muscle contraction and extension, your mind can recruit more muscle fibers and thoroughly work the muscle.

Step 1: Perform each repetition by taking 2 seconds to lift the weight, 2 seconds to hold it in the contracted position and 2 seconds to lower it. The repetition cadence of the Two-Step Rep puts your muscles under tension for a total of 90 seconds per set. (6-second reps x 15 reps average = 90 seconds.) It keeps you from using momentum to assist the movement, therefore decreasing the potential for injury.

Step 2: Once you've used the Two-Step Rep technique for two or three weeks, you'll want to change your tempo so that your workouts don't get stale and your body continues to adapt to the changes it is going through. You could change to a 1-1-1 tempo, a 1-1-4 tempo, a 3-2-3 tempo or just about any tempo you can imagine. However, keep in mind your total Time Under Tension, or TUT. The TUT I've chosen for this program (about 90 seconds per set) is ideal for strength endurance and fat burning. But if you want to grow really huge muscles, you'll want to lower your total TUT to between 40 and 70 seconds per set. If you want to increase your strength without increasing much in size, choose a cadence that puts your TUT under 20 seconds per set, such as five reps of 1-1-1.

EXERCISE:

The Muscle Math Counting Technique for High-Repetition Sets

Numbers of reps, numbers of sets, how many seconds between sets—it can all feel like a big math class some days. As you will soon see, the *Mind Over Muscle* routines have bouts of great intensity, where your repetition range will sometimes reach up to 25 repetitions! This is no easy feat. But here's a powerful way to trick your mind—and your body—into doing the repetitions you want.

Step 1: During this practice, break your ultimate repetition number into smaller repetition ranges. For example, if your repetition number goal is 25 repetitions, count in 4 blocks of 6 reps to get to 24 (and then do 1 for good luck for 25).

(**Please note:** *If you don't successfully reach your intended rep range, don't fret. The fact that you are using this high intensity protocol will have a positive effect on your body even if you only reached the 20th repetition.*)

Step 2: If you *still* didn't reach your goal number of repetitions, this may be due to reasons other than being bad in math: fatigue, for instance, or loss of concentration. When this happens, take 10 seconds to catch your breath, breathe deeply and then go right back to your exercise; starting from wherever you left off. For example, if you were shooting for 50 repetitions and using the Muscle Math exercise, your goal is to complete approximately six 8-repetition blocks. Let's say, in this case, that you were only able to reach the third block successfully, which means you've accomplished a grand total of 24 repetitions. Take a 10 second break and go right back and do another three blocks of 3 repetitions. If you can only do 1 block at a time, that's fine, too. Take your 10-second rest between each block.

Remember to think to yourself that your next block of repetitions is actually "the first set." Soon you will be done

with the total repetitions for that given set, thanks to Muscle Math-ing it all the way.

EXERCISE:

The Full Body Tension Technique for High-Load Strength

This mind-to-muscle technique is primarily used during compound exercises like the bench press, shoulder press, squat, or dead lift. The idea is to recruit every muscle in the body in order to increase your strength. The additional supporting muscles enable a lifter to take on heavier weights than usual while still keeping a safe body posture.

Step 1: To perform the Full Body Tension technique, get your body and weight into the pre-rep position. For a squat or dead lift, this means your knees are bent and your back is straight and you are about to exert the effort required to lift the weight. For bench or shoulder presses, this means the weight is against or almost against your chest and you are about to press it toward the sky.

Step 2: Once in position, clear your mind and focus on your muscles. Begin by squeezing the bar or handle and, muscle by muscle, work your way up (or down) your arms, consciously tensing every muscle as you go. When you reach the shoulders, begin tensing or contracting your chest muscles, back muscles, abdominals and glutes. With every new muscle you tense, you are continuing to keep previous muscles tense.

Step 3: Now work your way down the legs—especially for squats and dead lifts. It may seem like a lot of extra work at first, but with practice it will only take three seconds or less to complete the tensing part of this technique.

Step 4: When your body is solid as a rock, inhale and hold it—keeping your abs and glutes contracted especially tight. Now press through your legs for squats and dead lifts and through your arms for presses. Visualize the strength of the peripheral muscles (the muscles that aren't the primary target for the exercise) flowing into the primary muscles (like streams into a river) and grind your way to the full extension or contraction (like a wave crashing over the shore).

Step 5: Next take a short, shallow breath and begin a controlled descent under the same full-body tension. In the relaxed position take a deep breath or two while you release the tension throughout your body. For squats, take your breath in the standing position rather than the squatting position.

Step 6: Now begin tensing for your next rep.

EXERCISE:
The Screw Tension Technique
for Extreme Strength

The Screw is a combination of tension and visualization techniques that turn your arms or legs into mammoth pistons. Again, the object here is to recruit more muscle fibers than normal in order to lift heavier than usual weights. As always, practice with your usual load before trying heavier loads.

Step 1: When pressing a weight, especially a barbell, inhale while the weight is in the pre-rep position (close to your chest) and tense up all the muscles in your arms, back, and chest.

Step 2: As you go to press the weight up, make an isometric turning motion against the bar or handle as if you are going to "screw" the weight up with your arms. Your right arm will screw clockwise, and your left arm will screw counterclockwise, as if you were going to bring your elbows to your sides. Note that your elbows are not actually going to move much—the screwing motion is an isometric contraction.

The legs work basically the same way, but you are screwing them into the ground to press the weight up. Again, the right screws clockwise and the left counterclockwise.

EXERCISE:
The Flushing Technique
for Superior Muscle Size

This mind-to-muscle technique prepares your muscles to increase dramatically in size. (Ladies, if you want your muscles to remain sleek and trim, you may want to skip this technique.) The technique of "flushing" causes large amounts of blood to fill the capillaries around muscles and triggers creation of lactic acid. Both of these processes help stimulate growth in muscle size.

Step 1: Flushing comes into play on the final rep of a set and can be used with any muscle and any exercise. Once you've reached the last rep in a set that you can do with good form, begin another rep but stop before you complete the full contraction or extension. It can be halfway, a quarter- or three-quarters of the way to the full movement; it doesn't matter.

Step 2: Now, hold the weight at that stopping point for about 10 seconds and feel the muscles contract as they literally flush with blood. It's not just about holding the position as long as you can; it's about concentrating on the muscle and getting it under your conscious control.

If you're looking for large, sculpted muscles, include flushing as a regular part of your program. Each workout session, pick one exercise and use the flushing technique after the last rep of each set. Try to hold the second set's flush longer than the first set's flush, and hold the third set's flush longer than that, and so on.

EXERCISE:
Rockin Reps

Rockin Reps is based on the Two-Step Rep you've already learned. But instead of you counting how long each segment of a rep will take, you'll use the music to gauge your timing.

Step 1: Choose a song you like with a steady, well-defined tempo. Count out the beats (1, 2, 1, 2) to make sure it is not too fast or too slow.

Step 2: Perform each repetition by taking 2 counts of music to lift the weight, 2 counts to hold it in the contracted position and 2 counts to lower it.

For more information about Rockin Reps, please visit www.rockinreps.com.

EXERCISE:
Yoga Poses

Yoga, a 5000-year-old mind-body practice from India, has become mainstream in the United States. There are many different styles of yoga, but most start with the same basic poses. There are many books, DVDs, and classes that can teach you more about yoga, but here are a few poses to give you a taste of this ancient but vibrant practice. Hold each pose for several minutes. Make your mind still and concentrate on your breath.

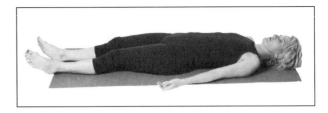

Corpse Pose: Lie on your back and let your arms and legs fall gently alongside your body. Turn your head from side to side. Then stretch out, breathing deeply and slowly from your abdomen.

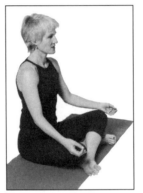

Easy Pose: Sit down and cross your legs, placing your feet below your knees. Clasp your hands around your knees. Keep your head and body straight.

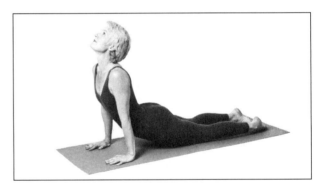

Cobra Pose: Lie on your belly, while your head rests on your lower arms. Raise your forehead, look upwards and stretch your hands backwards. Let your head falls a little backwards towards your back. Straighten your arms and turn them a little inward. Keep your shoulders relaxed, and breathe deeply and slowly.

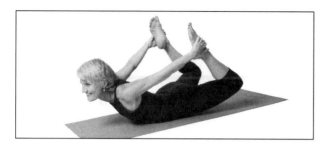

Bow Pose: Lie on your belly and let your forehead rest on your lower arms. Bend both legs and grab your ankles. Raise your head, look upwards. and stretch backward from your chin and your neck. Let your weight rest on your stomach and not on your pelvis. Raise your knees further by pulling your ankles with your hands. Rock back slightly as you inhale, and rock forward slightly as you exhale.

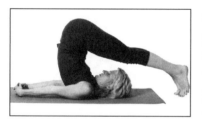

Plough Pose: Lie on your back with your legs stretched in front of you. Lift your hips and back off the floor, and bring your legs up, over, and behind your head. Bend your knees towards your shoulders, and clasp your arms behind you.

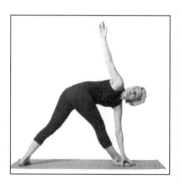

Triangle Pose: Stand with your feet three to four feet apart, and turn your right foot out slightly. Bend forward and put your left hand beside right foot, keeping your lower back straight. With your back straight and your left hip stretched backward, look at a point on the ground and breathe in and out quietly. Twist your chest to the right and stretch your right arm upward. Then twist your head to the right, look upward along your outstretched arm.

EXERCISE:
Sun Salutation

The Sun Salutation is a series of 12 poses that flow into one another, and help improve strength and flexibility. There are several variations on the Sun Salutation; this is one of the simplest.

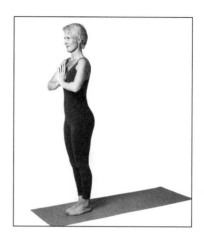

Step 1: Stand with your hands in prayer position. This is the Mountain Pose.

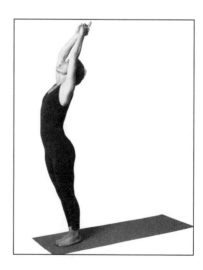

Step 2: As you inhale, raise your arms overhead and reach slightly backwards. Keep your hands clasped together.

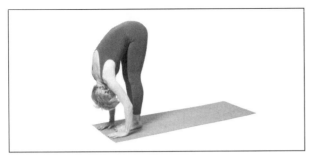

Step 3: As you exhale, bend forward and touch your hands to your feet.

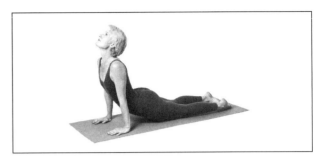

Step 7: As you inhale, stretch forward, bend back, and straighten your arms. This is the Cobra Pose.

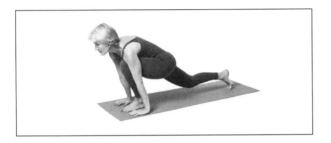

Step 4: As you inhale, step your right leg back into a lunge.

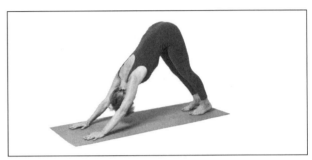

Step 8: As you exhale, curl your toes under, press down into your heels, and lift your hips. This is the Downward Dog Pose.

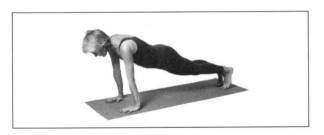

Step 5: As you exhale, step your left leg back into a push-up or plank position. Keep your spine and legs in a straight line.

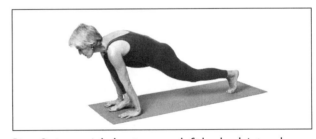

Step 9: As you inhale, step your left leg back into a lunge.

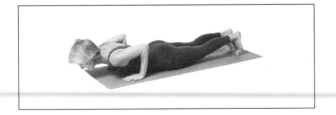

Step 6: Holding your breath, lower yourself slowly to the floor, first with your knees, then chest, then forehead.

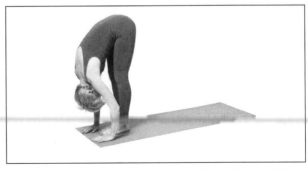

Step 10: As you exhale, bring your left leg forward, then bend forward and touch your hands to your feet.

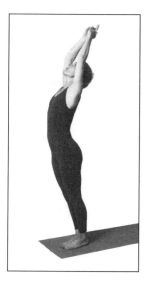

Step 11: As you inhale, raise your arms overhead and reach slightly backwards. Keep your hands clasped together.

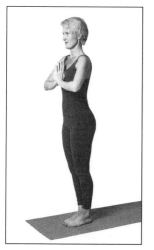

Step 12: As you exhale, come back into your starting position.

For more information about yoga, please visit www.trivelltechnique.com.

We often think of exercise and working out in active terms: fit, buff, amped, revved up, turned on, jazzed. But sometimes less is more, and for every yin there must be a yang. Case in point: in order to fully achieve results your body must rest. Without rest your body—and mind—will falter.

No matter how active you are, no matter how energetic your workouts, you must be just as vigilant about rest and recuperation to allow for even more active, energetic workouts in the future.

When you rest, you are not only resting your body, but also your mind. So mindful recovery is needed, and in fact will be one of the most important aspects of the program. To that end we will discuss the following in this chapter:

• The Day After—Rest Days
• Injury Prevention
• Your Mindset—Believe & Achieve

The Day After

When we exercise we need to remember that "the after" is just as important as "the during." When lifting weights, in particular, recovery is just as important as are reps. Therefore the day after a workout can be particularly useful in rebuilding and repairing muscles torn during the previous day's workouts.

This is an oft-overlooked part of the exercise regimen, for through the popular media and some not-so-prudent "experts" we have been taught that faster is better, "no pain, no gain," and that rest is for the weak or inexperienced. However, nothing could be further from the truth.

When you lift weights you are actually breaking down tissue and, through rebuilding, making that same tissue stronger for next time. This is how we grow stronger, bigger, faster, better. This is not a destructive thing; far from it. This tearing/rebuilding pattern is quite natural and in fact beneficial to keep the body healthy, vital, and strong. When you do this, however, your body needs to rest to fully benefit from the rebuild. After all, your body is still working; even if you're not!

Chapter 5:

Mindful Recovery

Work Hard At Resting Well

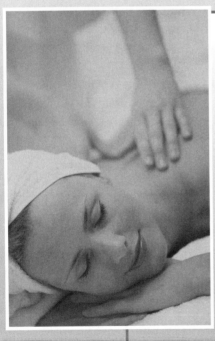

Beginners should take at least two days off during the week. For instance, as a beginner you will work out Monday, Wednesday, and Friday and will have a rest on Tuesday and Thursday. On Saturday and Sunday the beginner will consider doing a light workout just to get the muscles loose and moving and to stay active so that you're not stiff as a board for that Monday workout.

A more advanced person will alternate days of heavy workouts and days of light workouts. The light workouts will be the resting day, but since they are advanced in their habits they will have to do more on their days off. A complete day off is still important, so even people in the advanced bracket should take the rest seriously.

On your resting days you need to practice patience. This can be hard for some people, particularly considering the success you might already be having on this program. If you are unhappy with your results just keep in mind that they are coming. Do not exercise on your day off. You may do stretching, but do not exercise. By breaking your routine and schedule you will do more harm than good. By being patient and allowing your body to create the results when it is ready you are essentially recognizing that your body will build its physique when it is time. Do not rush recovery because you will realize a decrease in results and possibly hurt yourself.

Now, since I recognize that off days might be a challenge for many of you I have a few suggestions for how to fill them. If you just can't get enough of the gym on your off days, go there but don't exercise. Dress for a workout, but take a tour instead. Go into rooms and areas you haven't yet explored. Check out the bulletin board for classes that might interest you or talk to some instructors if they have a minute or two. Sometimes in the hustle and bustle of our workouts, we focus only on the machines we use, ignoring (often to our detriment) all the amenities and opportunities a modern gym affords.

After you've toured the gym, check out your local sporting goods store for various pieces of equipment you might be able to use at home, such as jump ropes, treadmills, the latest running shoes, etc. Either of these ideas should be more than enough to satisfy your "fitness fix" but can still qualify as off days so that your body can repair itself and your on days can be even more beneficial and satisfying.

EXERCISE:

Mindful Recuperation

Your days off are also a good time to do some "mindful exercises" (don't be confused by the name, your mind can exercise while your body is at rest).

Step 1: To begin, you can meditate as a way to better facilitate mindful rest. A feeling of peacefulness and

tranquility is the best setting for both your mind and muscles to repair from yesterday's rigors and prepare for tomorrow's.

Step 2: Next, you can use the visualization techniques we've discussed to create healthful, pleasing images of your muscle fibers repairing themselves or even growing larger from your efforts. Whatever you do, be careful not to compartmentalize your knowledge; what's good for your body is good for your mind, and vice versa.

Injury Prevention

"Walk it off." "No pain, no gain." These are just some of the erroneous suggestions made by insensitive bystanders when one experiences an injury. Don't believe them. An injury can be more than a temporary setback, especially if you ignore the pain and/or symptoms and put additional stress, wear, or tear on an already injured muscle, tendon, or limb. Take injuries seriously and remember that a week off to heal properly is better than a month off to heal improperly!

One of the most common injuries for a person working out with weights is for the joints to become sore. This is because a strain is put on the bones and cartilage during the repeated stress of extensions and contractions during repeated reps, sets, and workouts. In order to relieve this situation, there are some remedies that you can take. Glucosamine and gelatin have been found to soothe joint pain by stimulating cartilage growth. The best way to get these chemicals in your body is not through some hi-tech injection or expensive supplements, but through good, old-fashioned Jell-O. So, add Jell-O to your diet in order to prevent any joint or bone injuries.

Another way to prevent injuries is by proper stretching. Stretching is one of the most important and beneficial parts of any exercise program, but it's also one of the most frequently ignored elements by thousands who participate in regular physical workouts. Part of this is due to our busy schedules—we're in a hurry and when time is crunched, stretching seems to be the first to go. This is also due in part to the misconception that stretching is only required for some exercise, such as jogging or cardio. However, any exercise where the muscles, joints, and cartilage are engaged—i.e. ALL exercise—should be preceded by a reasonable amount of low-impact stretching.

For more information on recovery and ways to enhance your results, please visit www.mycustom-workout.com/recoverysecrets.

For best results, engage in a stretching routine that targets the entire body (legs, back, arms, groin, torso) but concentrate on the areas that you use primarily in your regular physical activities.

Do about five minutes of jogging in place before beginning to stretch. Stretching cold muscles increases the risk of injury to muscles, ligaments and delicate joints.

Since we're debunking a lot of myths in this chapter, let's pop one last kernel: when it comes to stretching, more is not always better. One last thing for you to remember is that you should never *overstretch*. If you stretch too much then you are actually stretching ligaments, not muscles, and increasing the likelihood of injury. So if a stretch hurts, stop.

EXERCISE:
Mindful Healing

An effective way to increase the healing power of the mind is through the release of endorphins, the brain's own painkillers. So what is the most effective way to release endorphins? Many studies have suggested basic imagery where the brain actually imagines healing the symptoms. This is similar to other techniques discussed throughout this book, but in this case the technique involves healing the body instead of building the body. For instance, one study had patients "visualize their white blood cells as powerful 'sharks' swimming through the bloodstream attacking weak, confused germs." (Ornstein and Sobel) If you're sore or have strained yourself after a workout, you can use a similar technique:

Step 1: Visualize that your muscles are strings, and that one of the strings is currently "weak."

Step 2: Now imagine that you are making more and more strings around the weak string and connecting them all together to make a larger and stronger string. After all, this is what you are doing when building your muscles. Your mind will thus release endorphins to help with the pain and further will allow your body to work to repair itself just as it does with disease.

Your Mindset

What you believe to be true—your mindset—is often more important than what is true. Exercise is as much about your mindset as it is your physical appearance, skill, or acuity. Many of the most physically fit people I've worked with began just like you are now, one day at a time. Many of them never thought they'd participate in competitions, run a marathon, or be in better shape than they were in high school, but now they do all of the above and so much more. This isn't necessarily because they're superior athletes; it's because they believe they can.

What you believe to be true will help you achieve your results. I'm not going to imply that you can "think yourself thin" or "flap your wings and fly," but I do want you to understand that your mindset can produce incredible results that you never thought possible in a million years.

Your mind is a strange thing because it can be the most important tool in helping you meet your goals, and at the same time it can be the biggest factor in sabotaging your efforts. The deciding factor in which way your mind goes—success or failure, triumph or defeat—lies in another bodily organ: your heart. So "take heart," for the following exercises will help you believe in yourself and therefore achieve your results.

EXERCISE:
Build a Positive Mindset

Step 1: First, you must always find a positive to take away with you every time you workout. Even if the positive is only that you did not give up, you still must make that fact a success in your work out. For instance, let's say that you had a bad workout and dropped in the amount of weight you were lifting, could not do all of the repetitions you wanted to, etc. In short, it was a crummy workout all the way around. Now, you *could* see this as a negative and a regression in your training, or you could see this as a positive in that you tried your best and never gave up. So what if it was a bad workout? At least you showed up.

Step 2: Avoid comparing yourself to others. Comparing yourself to others is a sure route to disappointment. Others we might compare ourselves to have been working out for years. Even if we start exercising on the same day as someone else who seems to have better results,

there are many reasons why they might "seem" more in shape than we are. Maybe they're 10 years younger, maybe they have a personal trainer, or maybe their metabolism is higher. Our only true litmus test is our positive feelings toward what we're accomplishing, even if it doesn't seem that "accomplished" at the time. Every day we move forward is another we're not left behind. Just picking up this book and reading it is perhaps more than you did last month or even all of last year. Now you're finally doing it. You have come so far I'm positive that any setback can now be met with perseverance, pride, and positivity.

Step 3: To help reinforce your positive feedback, you should also build an encouraging support team. Your friends will help you maintain your belief in yourself and encourage your best performance. By the same token, avoid friends or coaches that try to downplay your achievements, because this will only instill doubt in your mind.

Step 4: Perspective can be a great positivity builder. By stepping back from the situation from time to time—going to a new gym, going at a different time of day, running a different mile than you normally do, taking the scenic route instead of the most direct one—you can often see things in a different light. Believe it or not, even success can become routine. Sometimes we have poor workouts because we're bored, restless, or at a plateau. Shaking things up a little can often have a decidedly positive effect.

PART
TWO:

The Muscle

Now it is time to provide you with all the tools, the training, the technique, the tips and yes, the pictures, you need to design, implement, and begin your very own personal fitness program.

Here are all the latest *Mind Over Muscle* exercises, tried and tested (and even modeled) by myself and my students, specifically for this program. While some of them may look familiar at first—there are only so many ways to portray a bicep curl or squat thrust—the directions, reps, sets and overall philosophy for applying the *Mind Over Muscle* values to each exercise will soon be readily apparent.

For convenience and ease, you'll find the physical exercise (the muscle) listed first, followed immediately by the mental exercises (the mind). In no way does this imply that the muscle is more important than the mind. The mind will play a key part in building the muscle, and you should do both exercises at the same time. A strong mental edge usually comes from a firm grasp of the physical fundamentals. Master your technique and form and you'll find that the mental techniques will become much more powerful for you.

In keeping with the holistic emphasis of these muscle techniques, remember always to fall back on the Zone-Tone if you're having difficulty completing any of these exercises, or even feeling stale or unmotivated to complete a set or rep. It's a very useful exercise and one that I think you'll find invaluable as you begin to train in earnest. Also, I suggest that you use the Two-Step Rep or Rockin Reps technique to keep your tempo steady and your mind focused with each of these exercises. Remember: these mental techniques are not tricks but tools to help your mind feel better, stronger, and more positive about continuing to do something that's not always pleasant or fun. By using this tool frequently through-out these exercises, you'll find the workouts more rewarding each time!

But before we get started, here are a few notes that apply to most every exercise:

1. There is usually more than one way to grip a bar or handle for each exercise. The various grips will target the muscle from different angles, and while I suggest a grip for each exercise that is likely to give you the best results, try different grips from time to time in order to fully develop your muscles. Here are the three most common grips:

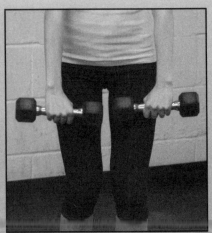

Pronated grip: palm faces behind you; your thumb points toward your body.

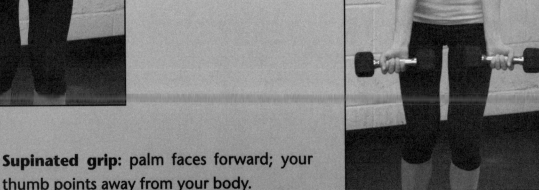

Supinated grip: palm faces forward; your thumb points away from your body.

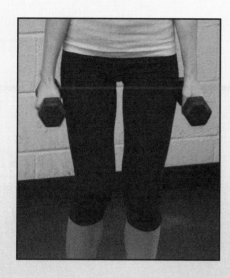

Neutral grip: palm faces your body; your thumb points forward.

(The muscles targeted by these grips varies according to the individual exercise.)

2. Choosing the right weight is important. You need to use a weight that allows you to perform an exercise with perfect form throughout the set. Most likely, that will be a weight that is lighter than you think. If you don't know what that weight is, start with a weight that seems ridiculously low and work your way up until you find the right weight. Once you are used to the exercise and can do all your sets with perfect form, you can increase your weight a bit each session. Do not increase the weight by more than 10% each week. Practicing perfect form with a light weight is easier than practicing with no weight, because the resistance helps you to feel the desired muscle being exercised, making it easier to isolate and stimulate that muscle. (This is another example of the "mind-to-muscle" connection.)

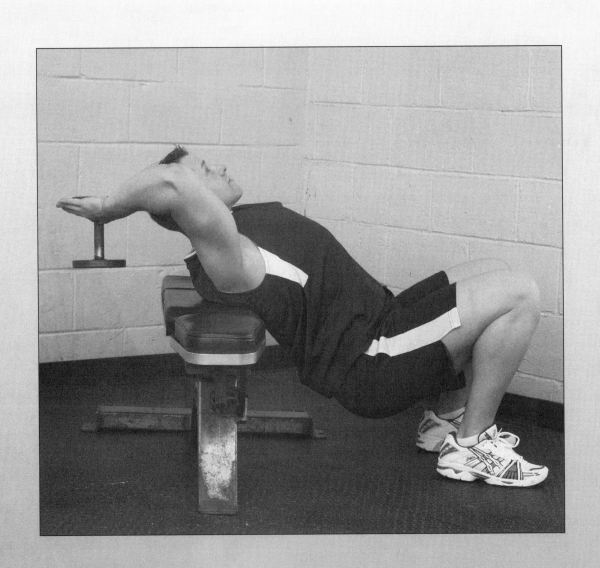

Chapter 6:

Chest and Back Exercises

Chest

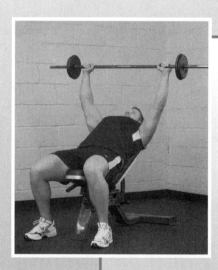

- Flat Barbell Bench Press

- Flat Dumbbell Bench Press

- Incline Barbell Bench Press

- Incline Dumbbell Bench Press

- Pushup

- Dumbbell Pullover

- Chest Dip

- Chair or Bench Dip

- Flat Dumbbell Fly

- Incline Dumbbell Fly

Flat Barbell Bench Press

PRIMARY TARGET MUSCLES: Middle Chest

NOTES: This exercise is the foundation for upper body strength because it incorporates all the major muscle groups, except for the back. Generally, a barbell will allow you to press more weight than dumbbells, making it a key exercise for upper body strength.

EXECUTION AND FORM

Step 1: With the barbell in the rack, lie back on the flat bench. Grip the bar with your hands slightly wider than shoulder width apart.

Step 2: Put your feet flat on the floor at the sides of the bench to help you with balance while lifting.

Step 3: Pinch your shoulder blades together against the flat bench so that it causes your chest to rise. You can imagine pinching a ball between your shoulder blades. This will take the shoulders out of the chest movement, allowing the chest to be the primary area working during the exercise.

Step 4: Unrack the bar and lower it in controlled fashion to within an inch of your chest. The bar should be over your sternum, not your collar bone or neck, so your elbows will not be quite perpendicular to your body.

Your forearms should be approximately perpendicular to the floor. If you are using heavy weights, have a partner assist with unracking the bar to avoid shoulder injuries.

Step 5: With the chest in its elevated position, the elbows out and wide, and the forearms perpendicular to the floor, tense up your chest muscles and prepare for the press.

Step 6: With your attention fully on your chest muscles, press the barbell up toward the ceiling. Before pressing, squeeze the barbell with your hands and keep that tension there throughout the exercise.

Step 7: As you reach the top of the exercise, be careful not to let the bar swing over your head. If it goes over your head, the weight transfers to the weaker anterior shoulder muscles and you risk serious injury.

Likewise, don't let the bar drift too far toward your pelvis where the weight again passes out of control of your chest muscles. Hold the final contraction.

Step 8: Once you've reached the top of the movement, begin lowering the weight while holding your proper postural alignment throughout the exercise.

Step 9: As the weight gets within an inch of your chest slowly begin to press the bar up again in a controlled, fluid motion, without using any momentum. Always stay focused and concentrate on the muscles being contracted.

Flat Barbell Bench Press

SECONDARY TARGET MUSCLES: **Anterior Deltoid, Triceps**

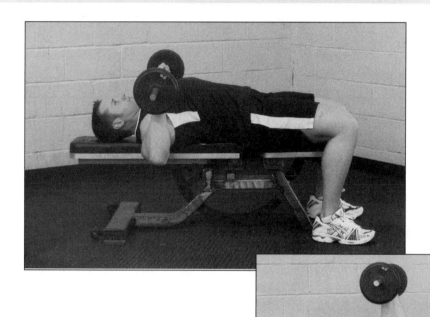

Mind Over Muscle Re-MIND-er:

Having trouble with the last rep in your set? Imagine there's an invisible person spotting you and they're there to help you through those last grueling inches to the top. They can pull as hard as you need them to. Or, try the Screw Tension Technique here, which will help you to drive the barbell up from the chest. Screw clockwise isometrically with your right hand and foot and counterclockwise with the left hand and foot.

Flat Dumbbell Bench Press

PRIMARY TARGET MUSCLES: Middle Chest

NOTES: Although you won't be able to press as much weight with dumbbells as you can a barbell, dumbbells allow for more stretch and isolation of the chest muscles. They also work each side of the chest independently, making strength imbalances less likely. With dumbbells, you'll need to work your way up from light weight so you can get accustomed to the movements without risking injury.

EXECUTION AND FORM

Step 1: Begin by sitting on the end of the bench with the dumbbells on your thighs. Thrust one leg up, leveraging the respective dumbbell up to your chest. Immediately thrust the second dumbbell upward with the other leg while simultaneously allowing momentum from the dumbbells to guide you back into the lying, supine position (flat, with your body facing the ceiling). Use your abdominal muscles to safely ease you into that position.

Step 2: Put your feet flat on the floor at the sides of the bench to help you with balance while lifting.

Step 3: Pinch your shoulder blades together against the flat bench so that it causes your chest to rise. You can imagine pinching a ball between your shoulder blades. This will take the shoulders out of the chest movement, allowing the chest to be the primary area working during the exercise.

Step 4: Position the dumbbells to the outside of your chest. Keep your elbows wide and the forearms perpendicular to the floor. Find a position that is wide enough to be comfortable and not so wide as to redirect the force to the shoulders. The wider you go beyond a comfortable position, the more likely you are to redirect the force of the weight onto the shoulders rather than the pecs. Even worse, when you widen your arms excessively when pressing a heavy or even moderate weight, you are actually causing the outer pectoral muscle to tear.

Step 5: With the chest in its elevated position, the elbows out and wide, and the forearms perpendicular to the floor, tense up your chest muscles and prepare for the press.

Step 6: With your attention fully on your chest muscles, press the dumbbells up toward the ceiling.

Step 7: As you reach the top of the exercise, you can either touch the dumbbells together or press them straight up like a barbell press. You can play around with different positions at the top of the movement as you may get a better muscle contraction by varying the dumbbell positions. The most important thing is to get the most intense contraction possible. You can do this by simply touching the dumbbells together and squeezing, or you can turn the dumbbells slightly inward at the top of the movement, allowing for a more controlled and isolated contraction. Hold this contraction.

Step 8: After you've reached the top of the movement, begin lowering the weight while holding your proper postural alignment throughout the exercise.

Step 9: As the weights get level with your chest, slowly begin to press the dumbbells up again in a controlled, fluid motion, without using any momentum. Always stay focused and concentrate on the muscles being contracted. If you don't have any type of shoulder injuries or muscle

Flat Dumbbell Bench Press

SECONDARY TARGET MUSCLES: Anterior Deltoid, Triceps

impingement, you may allow the dumbbells to lower to a comfortable stretch where the dumbbells are parallel with your chest. Always make sure that you stay in control of the dumbbells and maintain this control throughout the exercise.

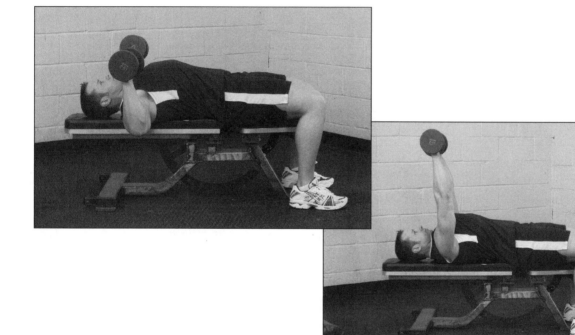

Mind Over Muscle Re-MIND-er

Don't rush your reps. Perform each repetition properly, with good form on both the lifting phase (concentric) and on the lowering phase (eccentric) of the weight. Keeping perfect form and technique is much more important than just trying to do all of your intended repetitions for a set. If you find yourself becoming sloppy, using too much momentum and losing form, stop the exercise, lower the weight and begin again. Really engage your mind/muscle connection and feel and think about each rep to stimulate the intended muscles to their maximum potential.

Incline Barbell Bench Press

PRIMARY TARGET MUSCLES: Upper Chest

NOTES: The incline barbell bench press targets the upper chest muscles and will give you that "big chest" look. Typically, you will not be able to use as much weight on the incline bench press as you would on the flat bench press because you are isolating a smaller section of the chest.

EXECUTION AND FORM

Step 1: With the barbell in the rack, lie back on the bench with the backrest set at a 45- to 60-degree angle. Grip the bar with your hands slightly wider than shoulder width apart.

Step 2: Put your feet flat on the floor at the sides of the bench to help you with balance while lifting.

Step 3: Pinch your shoulder blades together and downward against the back rest so that it causes your chest to rise. You can imagine pinching a ball between your shoulder blades. This will take the shoulders out of the chest movement, allowing the chest to be the primary area working during the exercise.

Step 4: Unrack the bar and lower it in controlled fashion to within an inch of your chest. The bar should be over your sternum, not your collar bone or neck, so your elbows will not be quite perpendicular to your body. Your forearms should be approximately perpendicular to the floor. If you are using heavy weights, have a partner assist with unracking the bar to avoid shoulder injuries.

Step 5: With the chest in its elevated position, the elbows out and wide, and the forearms perpendicular to the floor, tense up your chest muscles and prepare for the press. Focus your attention and tensing on the upper pecs just below the collar bone.

Step 6: Before pressing, squeeze the barbell with your hands and keep that tension there throughout the exercise. Now press the bar straight up, with your focus on contracting the pectoral muscles.

Step 7: As you reach the top of the exercise, be careful not to let the bar swing over your head. If it goes over your head, the weight transfers to the weaker deltoid muscles and you risk serious injury. Likewise, don't let the bar drift too far toward your pelvis where the weight again passes out of control of your chest muscles. Hold the final contraction.

Step 8: Once you've reached the top of the movement, begin lowering the weight while holding your proper postural alignment throughout the exercise.

Step 9: Lower the weight to a level that is comfortable, making sure that the chest muscles hold the majority of the resistance.

Step 10: Slowly begin to press the weight up again in a controlled, fluid motion, without using any momentum. Always stay focused and concentrate on the muscles being contracted.

Incline Barbell Bench Press

SECONDARY TARGET MUSCLES: **Anterior Deltoid, Triceps**

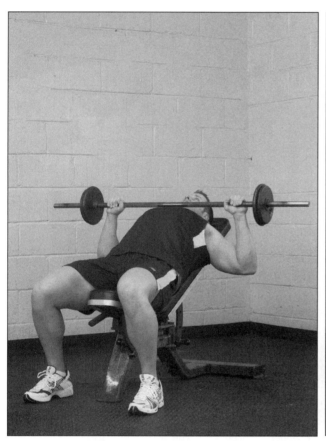 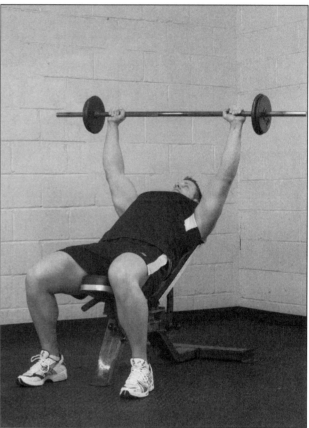

Mind Over Muscle Re-MIND-er

Specifically picture the upper pectoral muscles being activated. They are located along the top portion of your chest, just under the collar bone. Imagine that these muscles are colored red. During your exercise, consciously contract these muscles as your arms are being pushed up. The harder you push and contract these muscles, the brighter the color red gets. At the top of the movement (as your arms are at full extension), visualize your upper chest muscles shining bright red.

Incline Dumbbell Bench Press
(Pronated and Neutral Grips)

PRIMARY TARGET MUSCLES: Upper Chest

NOTES: The incline dumbbell bench press targets the upper chest muscles. When you develop the upper chest, it will give your entire chest the appearance of having a "shelf" like appearance. Typically, you will not be able to use as much weight on the incline bench press as you would on the flat bench press because you are isolating a smaller section of the chest. The dumbbell version can be performed with two grips: with palms facing forward or palms facing each other. For both grips, the movements are the same.

EXECUTION AND FORM

Step 1: Begin by sitting on the end of the bench with the dumbbells on your thighs. Thrust one leg up, leveraging the respective dumbbell up to your chest. Immediately thrust the second dumbbell upward with the other leg while simultaneously allowing momentum from the dumbbells to guide you back into an inclined position against the backrest, which should be set at a 45- to 60-degree angle. Use your abdominal muscles to safely ease you into that position.

Step 2: Put your feet flat on the floor at the sides of the bench to help you with balance while lifting.

Step 3: Pinch your shoulder blades together and downward against the backrest bench so that it causes your chest to rise. You can imagine pinching a ball between your shoulder blades. This will take the shoulders

out of the chest movement, allowing the chest to be the primary area working during the exercise.

Step 4: Position the dumbbells to the outside of your chest. Keep your elbows wide and the forearms perpendicular to the floor throughout the exercise movement. Find a position that is wide enough to be comfortable and not so wide as to redirect the force to the shoulders. The wider you go beyond a comfortable position, the more likely you are to redirect the force of the weight on to the shoulders rather than the pecs. Even worse, when you widen your arms excessively while pressing a heavy or even moderate weight, you are actually causing the outer pectoral muscle to tear.

Step 5: With the chest in its elevated position, the elbows out and wide and the forearms perpendicular to the floor, tense up your chest mus-

cles and prepare for the press. Focus your attention and tensing on the upper pecs just below the collar bone.

Step 6: With your attention fully on your upper chest muscles, press the dumbbells up toward the ceiling.

Step 7: As you reach the top of the exercise, you can either touch the dumbbells together or press them straight up like a bench press. You can play around with different positions at the top of the movement as you may get a better muscle contraction by varying the dumbbell positions. The most important thing is to get the most intense contraction possible. You can do this by simply touching the dumbbells together and squeezing, or you can turn the dumbbells slightly inward at the top of the movement, allowing for a more controlled and isolated contraction. Hold the final contraction.

Incline Dumbbell Bench Press
(Pronated and Neutral Grips)

SECONDARY TARGET MUSCLES: **Anterior Deltoid, Triceps**

Step 8: Once you've reached the top of the movement, begin lowering the weight while holding your proper postural alignment throughout the exercise.

Step 9: Lower the weight to a level that is comfortable, making sure that the chest muscles hold the majority of the resistance. If you don't have any type of shoulder injuries or muscle impingement, you may allow the dumbbells to lower to a comfortable stretch where the dumbbells are parallel with your chest. Always make sure that you stay in control of the dumbbells and maintain this control throughout the exercise.

Step 10: Slowly begin to press the weight up again in a controlled, fluid motion, without using any momentum. Always stay focused and concentrated on the muscles being contracted.

Mind Over Muscle Re-MIND-er:

When you're resting between sets, work on developing your mind-muscle connection by isometrically flexing one muscle at a time throughout your body. Start with one foot and work your way up that side of the body, across the shoulders and down the other side of the body until you've flexed every muscle that you know about. The trick is to flex each muscle in isolation, which will take some practice. It will probably take you several rest periods to complete the pattern.

Incline Dumbbell Bench Press
(Pronated and Neutral Grips)

SECONDARY TARGET MUSCLES: Anterior Deltoid, Triceps

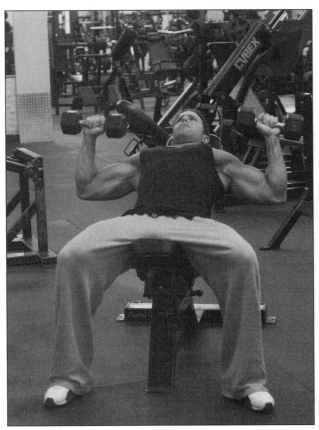

Pronated grip

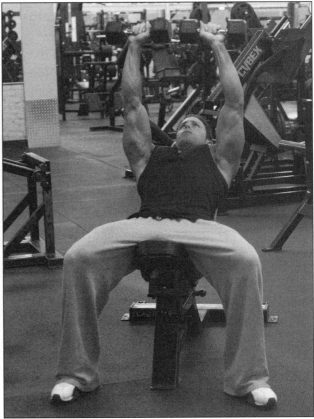

Incline Dumbbell Bench Press
(Pronated and Nuetral Grips)

PRIMARY TARGET MUSCLES: **Upper Chest**

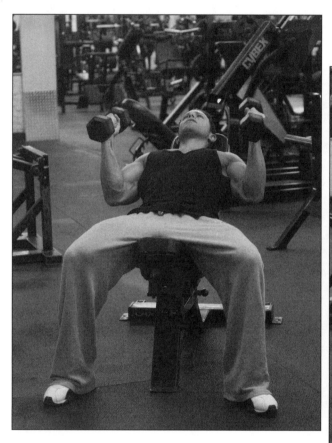

Neutral grip

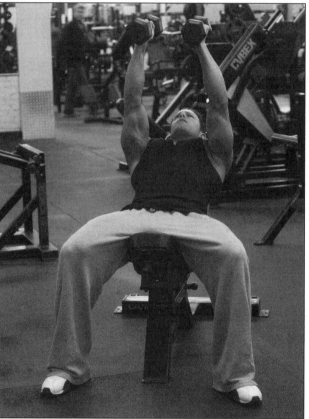

Pushup

PRIMARY TARGET MUSCLES: **Pectorals**

NOTES: Any time you don't have access to weight-lifting equipment, like when you're traveling, you can replace bench presses, dumbbell presses, and flies with simple pushups. Make pushups easier by elevating your hands higher than your feet or by doing them on your knees instead of your toes. To better simulate a dumbbell press, you can center your weight over one hand for half of the required reps and over the other hand for the remaining reps. This is not a one-arm push up; keep the second hand on the floor further from your body to help you balance. Elevate your feet onto a chair or other object to simulate the incline version of these exercises.

EXECUTION AND FORM

Step 1: Assume the standard pushup position with your body supported on only your toes and the palms of your hands. Start the exercise in the up position with your arms locked out. Your hands should be slightly wider than shoulder width apart with your fingers pointed forward, and your body should remain straight as a board throughout the exercise.

Step 2: Begin bending the elbows to lower your chest to the floor. Your chest should be the first and only part of your body to touch the floor. If your girth prevents you from touching your chest to the floor, try doing this exercise between two chairs by placing one hand on the seat of each chair and lowering yourself between them. Hold this contraction.

Step 3: Once your chest touches the floor, flex your pectoral muscles and push your body back up. If you're using the chair method mentioned above, stop lowering yourself when your chest reaches the level of the chair seats.

Pushup

SECONDARY TARGET MUSCLES: **Triceps, Shoulders**

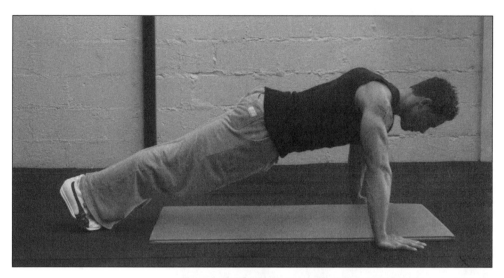

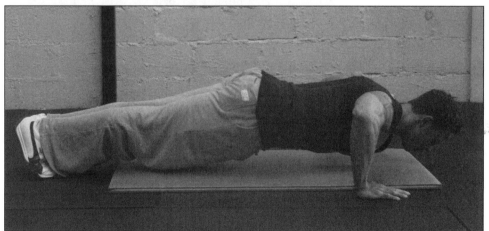

Mind Over Muscle Re-MIND-er:

Using Full Body Tension on this exercise will help you maintain a straight body throughout the exercise, give more support to your lower back, and keep the emphasis in the chest muscle.

Dumbbell Pullover

PRIMARY TARGET MUSCLES: Pectorals

NOTES: Although this exercise looks a little strange, it's great for the upper body. It does a great job of thickening the pectorals.

EXECUTION AND FORM

Step 1: Lie with your upper back across a flat bench, with a dumbbell in your hands.

Step 2: Ensure that your neck and your upper back are the only body parts resting on the bench.

Step 3: Stand a dumbbell on your chest and with two hands palm up, press it over your chest at arm's length. (Please ensure that the dumbbells you are using have their weights properly secured).

Step 4: Bring your focus and attention to your chest muscles and flex them. Imagine that your arms are a steel tower and your pecs are the cables that are keeping that tower vertical.

Step 5: Keep your arms straight as you slowly lower the dumbbell behind your head in an arc. Now your pectoral cables are slowly lengthening and allowing the weight to gradually pull down the steel tower of your arms—but remember, those arms are steel and straight! Ensure that your hips are not being raised as you lower the weight.

Step 6: When you reach the fully stretched position, hold the stretch. Now start reeling in that pectoral cable and raise the weight back up in an arc until you reach the starting position once again.

Dumbbell Pullover

SECONDARY TARGET MUSCLES: Triceps, Serratus Anterior

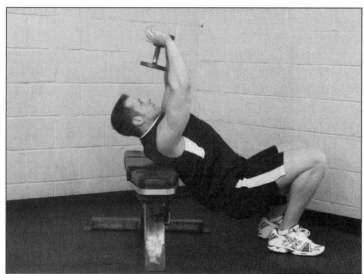

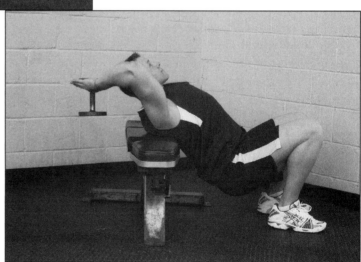

Mind Over Muscle Re-MIND-er:

When doing this particular exercise, think about the vertical pull and how the motion of this exercise stimulates the chest muscles differently from the other chest exercises.

Chest Dip

PRIMARY TARGET MUSCLES: Lower Chest

> **NOTES:** Never over-stress your muscles, tendons and ligaments. This exercise uses a parallel dip station. If this is difficult, you can put a chair behind you and put your toes on it so you can get a little help from your legs. Or try a weight assisted machine such as the Gravitron, which counterbalances a portion of your body weight. If you are working out in your home, I suggest you purchase an inexpensive dip unit from one of the sports-related retail chains or a wholesale fitness supply store. In a wholesale store, you can typically negotiate a lower price and the quality of the apparatus is usually much better. Look in your local yellow pages for the store nearest you.

EXECUTION AND FORM

Step 1: Place your hands on the parallel bars as you position yourself for postural alignment.

Step 2: The best way to align yourself is to raise yourself up onto the dip bars by locking out your arms. You will then align your body, starting with your head and moving down to your feet.

Step 3: While suspended in the top position of the exercise, your head will at first be level and looking straight ahead. You may find that bending your head slightly forward as you lower yourself will help you lean forward for increased muscle stimulation in the chest. You must constantly focus all of your attention on the chest muscles during this exercise as this will help increase the involvement of the chest muscles and keep you in the proper alignment.

Step 4: Bend your legs at the knees and hook your feet over one another. This will help keep your back arched forward for the ultimate involvement of the chest muscles.

Step 5: As you lower yourself from the lockout position, immediately begin to lean forward. The farther you lean forward, the more your chest muscles will work. Keep the elbows and arms away from your body, helping to better isolate the chest muscles and avoid recruiting the triceps. Lower yourself slowly while resisting your body weight all the way to the bottom position.

Step 6: Lower yourself until the backs of your arms are parallel or slightly beyond parallel with the floor. Remember, you should never go so low that you feel any chest or shoulder pain, or you could seriously injure yourself. Go to a point where you are comfortable and increase a little more the next session if needed.

Step 7: When you reach the bottom position, do not rest! Slowly, with a smooth transition, begin to press your body upward without using any momentum. Make sure that you maintain your postural alignment.

Step 8: As you begin pressing upward, make sure that all of your focus is once again directed to your chest muscles. This alone will help stimulate the triceps through increased muscle control. As you near the top of the motion, your goal is not to lock out the joint but to contract and squeeze the chest muscles as hard as you possibly can. It is important for the chest muscles to hold you in this position rather than lock out with the triceps or the elbow joints.

Step 9: Remember that there should be no rest at the top of the exercise after the contraction period. From that near-lock out position, once again

Chest Dip

SECONDARY TARGET MUSCLES: Triceps, Serratus

slowly lower yourself as you resist the weight of your body back to the bottom position. If you get to a point where your body weight is too light for the exercise, you may use a dip belt to hook some additional weight to your body, thus increasing the resistance. Please make sure that if you do use additional weight, you do so in small, incremental stages.

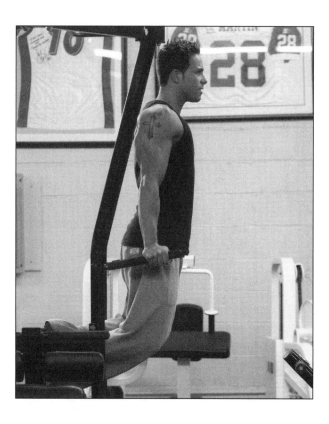 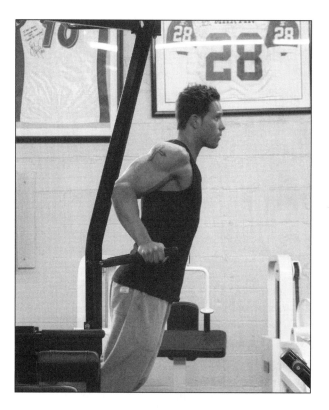

Mind Over Muscle Re-MIND-er:

Think about where you are feeling the muscle contractions. If it's in the triceps, you need to lean forward more over the handles to bring the chest into play more. You may also need to spread your elbows out wider. Remember to stay focused on the muscle contraction of the chest, no matter how exhausted you are, or how heavy the weight seems. The Screw Tension and Flushing Techniques also work wonders for this exercise.

Chair or Bench Dip

PRIMARY TARGET MUSCLES: Lower Chest

NOTES: If you don't have access to parallel bars for doing chest dips, you can do chair dips. These are performed just like chest dips, but you will use the backs of two chairs, a bench, or whatever furniture is available to you.

EXECUTION AND FORM

Step 1: Place your hands on the bench as you position yourself for postural alignment.

Step 2: The best way to align yourself is to raise yourself up onto the bench by locking out your arms. You will then align your body, starting with your head and moving down to your feet.

Step 3: While suspended in the top position of the exercise, your head will at first be level and looking straight ahead. You may find that bending your head slightly forward as you lower yourself will help you lean forward for increased muscle stimulation in the chest. You must constantly focus all of your attention on the chest muscles during this exercise as this will help increase the involvement of the chest muscles and keep you in the proper alignment.

Step 4: Bend your legs at the knees and hook your feet over one another. This will help keep your back arched forward for the ultimate involvement of the chest muscles.

Step 5: As you lower yourself from the lockout position immediately begin to lean forward. The farther you lean forward, the more your chest muscles will work. Keep the elbows and arms away from your body, helping to better isolate the chest muscles and avoid recruiting the triceps. Lower yourself slowly while resisting your body weight all the way to the bottom position.

Step 6: Lower yourself until the backs of your arms are parallel or slightly beyond parallel with the floor. Remember, you should never go so low that you feel any chest or shoulder pain or you could seriously injure yourself. Go to a point where you are comfortable and increase a little more the next session if needed.

Step 7: When you reach the bottom position, do not rest! Slowly, with a smooth transition, begin to press your body upward without using any momentum. Make sure that you maintain your postural alignment.

Step 8: As you begin pressing upward, make sure that all of your focus is once again directed to your chest muscles. As you near the top of the motion, your goal is not to lock out the joint but to contract and squeeze the chest muscles as hard as you possibly can. It is important for the chest muscles to hold you in this position rather than lock out with the triceps or the elbow joints.

Step 9: Remember that there should be no rest at the top of the exercise after the contraction period. From that near-lockout position, once again slowly lower yourself as you resist the weight of your body back to the bottom position. If you get to a point where your body weight is too light for the exercise, use a dip belt to hook some additional weight to your body, thus increasing the resistance. Please make sure to do so in small, incremental stages.

Chair or Bench Dip

SECONDARY TARGET MUSCLES: **Triceps, Serratus**

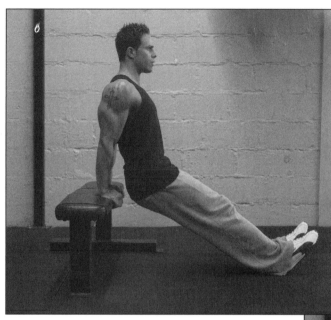

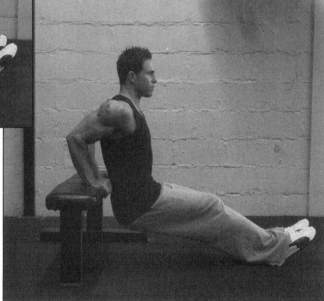

Mind Over Muscle Re-MIND-er:

When you're facing a set you expect to be difficult, tell yourself that you're full of energy, that your strength and stamina are phenomenal. In other words, turn a negative into a positive by psyching yourself up. Feel that energy and strength course through your body and become convinced that nothing in the world will stop you from finishing every last rep of that set. Nothing!

Flat Dumbbell Fly

PRIMARY TARGET MUSCLES: Middle Chest

NOTES: It might look as if this exercise is identical to the dumbbell bench press, but it is not. With the dumbbell press, you are straightening the elbow joint and utilizing horizontal adduction of the shoulder joints—the movement of bringing the arms together. The dumbbell fly must only incorporate the shoulder joints movement and not the elbow joints extension. The elbows must be locked into place for the exercise to be truly effective.

IMPORTANT: The further a weight gets from your body the heavier its actual load on the muscles is. With the fly, the weight gets nearly a full arm's length from the body, which effectively triples the weight. If you try to use the same dumbbells you used on the bench press, you will quickly lose control on the descent and could seriously damage muscles, tendons and ligaments and even possibly bones. I urge you to start light—really light—until you perfect the movement.

EXECUTION AND FORM

Step 1: You'll want to align your body exactly as you did with the dumbbell press, with your chest arched upward and your shoulder blades pinched together. But now you will have the palms of your hands facing each other instead of facing the wall in front of you.

Step 2: Begin by pressing the dumbbells to arms' length above you. Then lower the weights with control outward and downward until they are at approximately chest level. Your palms should face each other throughout the exercise. Keep your elbows nearly straight throughout the exercise.

Step 3: Inhale and focus on your chest muscles. Imagine your pecs contracting and drawing your arms together. Exhale and squeeze the dumbbells together in an upward arc while keeping your elbows locked at the same angle as when you started the move.

Step 4: As you arc the dumbbells upward, picture yourself hugging a tree. Imagine there is a tree between you and the dumbbells; you will be mimicking the exact motion of hugging it. This visualization technique will help keep you in the correct position to follow the arched movement. All of this will ensure that your chest muscles receive the most intense stimulation and contraction possible.

Step 5: As you reach the top of the movement, be sure to consciously contract the chest muscles as hard as you possibly can for maximum muscle stimulation.

Step 6: Begin lowering the weight while holding the proper alignment, technique, and form throughout the movement. As you reach the bottom of the movement, be sure not to let the back of the arms go too far below the level of your chest, as this could cause injury to the shoulder's rotator cuff.

Step 7: When you reach the bottom of the movement, slowly begin squeezing the dumbbells back upward in an arc again. Use a controlled, fluid motion, making sure you don't use momentum.

Flat Dumbbell Fly

SECONDARY TARGET MUSCLES: Anterior Deltoid

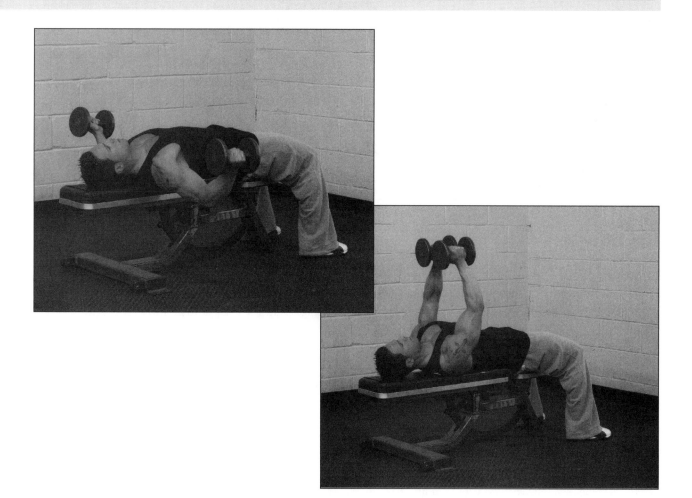

Mind Over Muscle Re-MIND-er:

Try doing this exercise just before doing the flat barbell bench press. This exercise, which does a great job of isolating the pectoral (chest) muscles, will "pre-exhaust" those muscles. When you hit the bench press, which is a compound exercise that doesn't isolate as well as the fly, the pectoral muscles will be fatigued, but the supporting muscles will be fresh and will force the pectorals to work harder. This will stimulate the pecs to their maximum potential for growth.

Incline Dumbbell Fly

PRIMARY TARGET MUSCLES: Upper Chest

NOTES: It might look as if this exercise is identical to the incline dumbbell bench press, but it is not. With the press, you are straightening the elbow joint and utilizing horizontal adduction of the shoulder joints—the movement of bringing the arms together. The fly must only incorporate the shoulder joints movement and not the elbow joints extension. The elbows must be locked into place for the exercise to be truly effective.

IMPORTANT: Start with less weight than you would use in a dumbbell press because you will have fewer muscles assisting the pectorals.

EXECUTION AND FORM

Step 1: You'll want to align your body exactly as you did with the incline dumbbell press, with your chest arched upward and your shoulder blades pinched together and downward. But now you will have the palms of your hands facing each other instead of facing the wall in front of you.

Step 2: Begin by pressing the dumbbells to arms' length above you. Then lower the weights with control outward and downward until they are at approximately chest level. Your palms should face each other throughout the exercise.

Step 3: Inhale and focus on your chest muscles. Imagine your pecs contracting and drawing your arms together.

Exhale and squeeze the dumbbells together in an upward arc while keeping your elbows locked at the same angle as when you started the move.

Step 4: As you arc the dumbbells upward, picture yourself hugging a tree. Make believe there is a tree between you and the dumbbells; you will be mimicking the exact motion of hugging it. This visualization technique will help keep you in the correct position to follow the arched movement. All of this will ensure that your chest muscles receive the most intense stimulation and contraction possible.

Step 5: As you reach the top of the movement, be sure to consciously contract the chest muscles as hard as you possibly can for maximum muscle stimulation.

Step 6: Begin lowering the weight while holding the proper alignment, technique and form throughout the movement. As you reach the bottom of the movement, be sure not to let the back of the arms go too far below the level of your chest, as this could cause injury to the shoulders' rotator cuff.

Step 7: When you reach the bottom of the movement, slowly begin squeezing the dumbbells back upward in an arc again. Use a controlled, fluid motion, making sure you don't use momentum.

Incline Dumbbell Fly

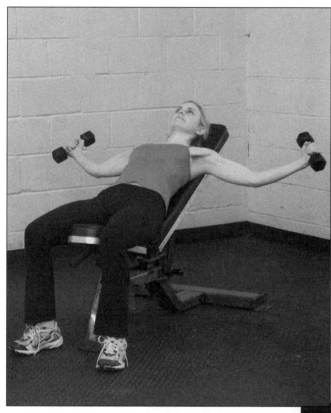

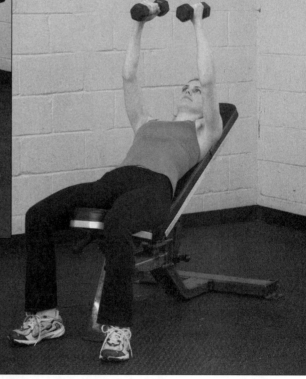

Mind Over Muscle Re-MIND-er:

When repetitions begin to get difficult, imagine that those dumbbells are magnetic. As you press them upward, feel the magnetic energy pull them up and together.

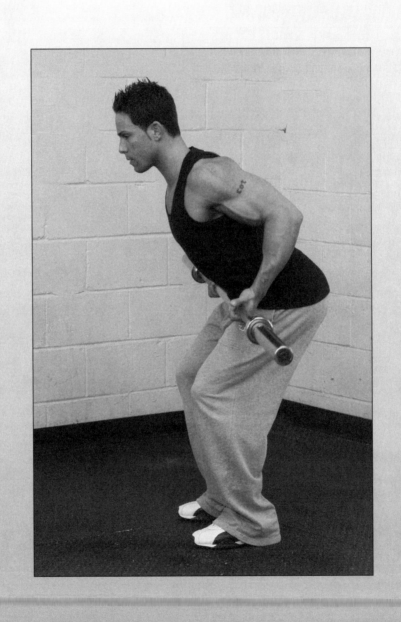

Back

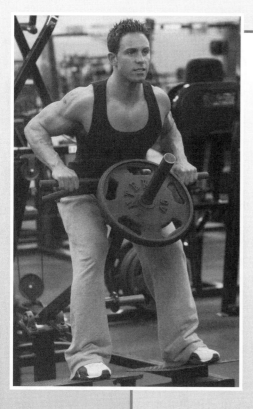

- Deadlift

- Towel Deadlift

- Barbell Row

- T-Bar Row

- T-Bar Machine Row

- Towel Row

- One-Arm Dumbbell Row

- Two-Arm Dumbbell Row

- Seated Machine Row

- Plate-Loaded One-Arm Row

- Low Pulley Row

- Standing High Pulley V-Bar Row

- Wide Grip Pullup

- Narrow Grip V-Bar Pullup

- Wide Grip Pulldown

- High Pulley V-Bar Pulldown

- Close Reverse Grip Pulldown

Deadlift

PRIMARY TARGET MUSCLES: Lower Back, Gluteals, Hamstrings

> **NOTES:** This exercise works more muscles than any other exercise. Sloppy form will injure your lower back, so be sure to pay close attention to the techniques described and study the illustrations carefully! Note that this is the only exercise in which you should fully lockout the body at the top of the movement. Attempting to hold the top position without locking out will put too much strain on the back.

EXECUTION AND FORM

Step 1: With a barbell on the floor in front of you, stand facing the bar with your feet shoulder width apart (or slightly less) and halfway under the bar.

Step 2: While still standing straight, look up to the ceiling and inhale deeply. As you descend to the bar, hold your breath, arch your lower back—don't round it—and squeeze your shoulder blades to hold your shoulders back. Make a point of pushing your butt back as if you were going to sit in a chair and keep your shins vertical.

Step 3: Remember to keep your eyes on the ceiling throughout the movement. This keeps your back aligned properly so that you will lift with your legs instead of your back. During the descent tighten up your entire body to keep alignment correct.

Step 4: Without looking at it, grip the bar with your hands slightly wider than shoulder width. Use an over-hand grip with one hand and an underhand grip with the other.

Step 5: Straighten your arms, tighten your abs and glutes and remember: you are still holding your breath. Squeeze the bar with your hands and turn your focus to your legs. Tighten up your legs—imagine them as huge, coiled springs ready to launch you to the moon. PRESS THROUGH YOUR HEELS TO PUSH THE FLOOR AWAY FROM YOU. Do not pull on the barbell! Pulling uses your back and arms, which is the way to get injured. Push with your legs and let the barbell follow.

Step 6: Stay tight throughout the movement. Envision your legs as giant, hydraulic pile drivers burrowing into the ground. Your back is a crane: straight and strong. Your arms are cables, just carrying the load.

Step 7: Near the top of the lift give your hips a slight thrust forward and throw back your shoulders to com-pletely straighten your body. Keep your chest high but DO NOT LEAN BACK. You are still looking at the ceiling. You are still holding your breath.

Step 8: At the top, you can take a shallow breath before you lower the bar to the ground.

Step 9: To lower the bar, keep your back straight and push your butt back, bending at the hips. Do not attempt to control the descent of the bar too much; doing so puts dangerous strain on your back. However, don't purposefully drop the bar either. Remember to stay on your heels and continue looking at the ceiling.

Step 10: Before doing your next rep, let go of the bar and stand up. Re-align your posture from the beginning and descend to grab the bar again. If you don't stand up between sets, your form is guaranteed to deteriorate, which will likely result in injury.

Deadlift

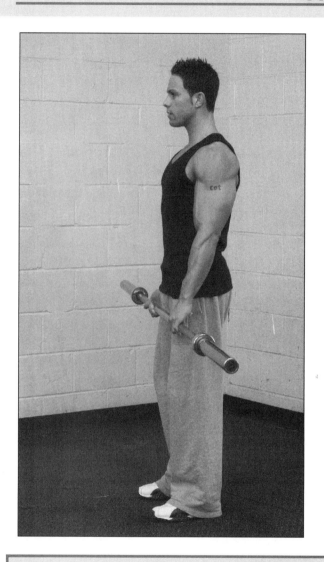
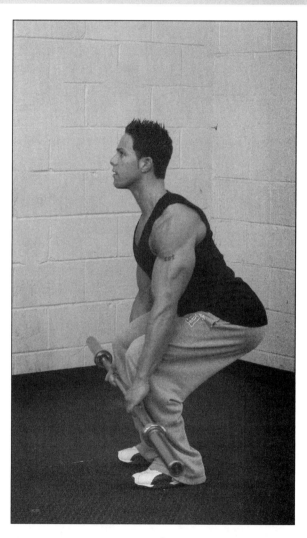

Mind Over Muscle Re-MIND-er:

This exercise requires full concentration and focus to stay tight and straight. Your mind needs to be fully engaged with this exercise, making sure that all of your muscles are assisting in the movement. Most importantly, you need to be constantly aware of your back and keep it in proper alignment. The Full Body Tension technique is ideal for the deadlift, because it contracts every muscle in your body, which keeps it locked in alignment.

Towel Deadlift

PRIMARY TARGET MUSCLES: Lower Back, Gluteals, Hamstrings

> **NOTES:** When you're traveling or don't have access to a barbell or deadlift machine, deadlifts can be done isometrically using a towel rolled lengthwise or a rope. Since this is a form of isometric exercise, in which there is no joint movement, hold the contraction for a total of 6 seconds rather than using the Two-Step Rep method.

EXECUTION AND FORM

Step 1: Lay the towel or rope out straight on the floor and stand centered on it with your feet approximately shoulder width apart. Make sure the ends of the towel or rope are sticking out beyond your feet enough for you to grab them.

Step 2: Assume the position for a standard bent-knee deadlift and grab an end of the towel in each hand.

Step 3: Straighten your arms, tighten your abs and glutes and remember: you are still holding your breath. Squeeze the towel with your hands and turn your focus to your legs. Tighten up your legs and press through your heels to push the floor away from you. Stay tight throughout the movement.

Step 4: Near the top of the lift imagine that your hips thrust forward and your shoulders are thrown back. But do not actually do this movement.

Step 5: At the top, take a shallow breath before you lower the towel to the ground and hold the isometric contraction.

Step 6: To lower the towel, keep your back straight and push your butt back, bending at the hips. Remember to stay on your heels and continue looking at the ceiling.

Step 7: Before doing your next rep, let go of the towel and stand up. Re-align your posture from the beginning and descend to grab the towel again.

Towel Deadlift

SECONDARY TARGET MUSCLES: Upper Back, Trapezius, Thighs

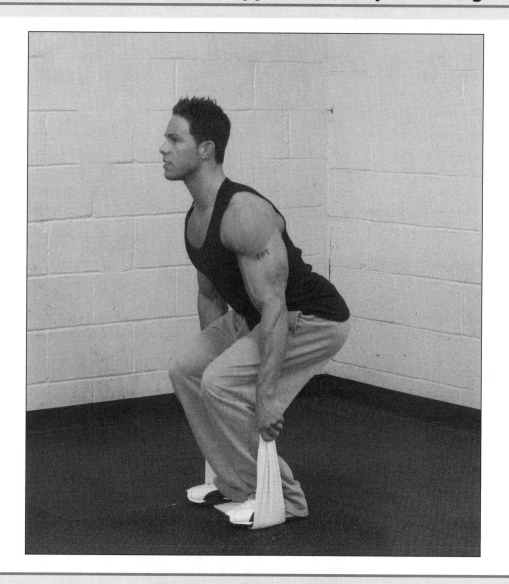

Mind Over Muscle Re-MIND-er:

Even though this exercise doesn't call for lifting heavy weight, imagine that you are moving a ton. Tell yourself how huge and strong you are. Exaggerate and marvel at how easy it is—kid's play even—and launch into the next rep. Building your confidence up this way will help you pull every ounce of effort out of your muscles.

Barbell Row

PRIMARY TARGET MUSCLES: Mid Back Latissimus Dorsi

> **NOTES:** Because the lower back is so vulnerable in this exercise, begin with a relatively light weight. With a few practice sessions, you will be able to perform the exercises with ease. I have noticed that once most clients learn to correctly execute the exercises they often make dramatic progress within a few days of beginning the program. People with lower back problems may be better off using dumbbells in place of a barbell or using the T-Bar Machine Row.

EXECUTION AND FORM

Step 1: Place a barbell in front of you on the ground, or on a rack at knee level.

Step 2: Align your feet about shoulder width apart. Make sure your knees are pointing directly in front of you with a slight bend throughout the movement.

Step 3: Bend over at the hips, making sure that your lower back is not slumped over. To make sure of this, squeeze or contract your abdominal and glute muscles while slightly arching your lower back. Do not bend over all the way, as this can injure the lower back. Your back should be parallel to the floor or slightly higher. But if you stand too upright, this positioning will not sufficiently activate the upper back muscles. You must be bent over to a degree where the elbows will naturally remain close to the body. At the same time, the back of the arms (triceps) follow a row-like movement, directly toward the ceiling.

Step 4: Pick up the bar using either a palms-down or a palms-up type of grip. The palms-down grip is recommended for beginners as with this grip the biceps are less involved. Advanced exercisers can use a palms-up grip, which will stress the lats more directly. As you pick up the bar, think about what muscles you are about to exercise. The lats are located on the outermost side of the back and are your focus point.

Step 5: Let the bar hang down. Keep the elbows slightly wider than shoulder width.

Step 6: Stick out your chest while slightly squeezing your shoulder blades together. This will position and keep your body in the proper alignment throughout the movement. Holding these alignment positions throughout the exercise will make sure stimulation remains in the back muscles.

Step 7: Contract the back muscles isometrically for the best results. Begin rowing the elbows up toward the ceiling, allowing the back of the arms (triceps) to lead the motion.

Step 8: Drive the elbows and back of the arms upward until the barbell is touching your lower belly and you are able to fully contract the back muscles. Imagine that there is an egg in the middle of your back. Your objective for each repetition, when the bar is being pulled to your belly, is to crack the egg with your back muscles

IMPORTANT: Your goal is not to touch the barbell to your chest, as this will put too much emphasis on the biceps.

Step 9: Keep your head up and looking straight ahead throughout the movement. This will help you keep your balance and make it easier to maintain the described position.

Step 10: Try to squeeze the muscles at the top of the movement. When doing this you are simultaneously learning to isolate those specific muscles. When you apply this technique

Barbell Row

SECONDARY TARGET MUSCLES: Lower Back, Rear Deltoids, Biceps

to an exercise, you are actually optimizing your training sessions through the increased muscle recruitment.

Step 11: Begin your descent with a slow and controlled movement. As you reach the bottom, slowly and smoothly begin the movement upward again without resting. Make sure that no momentum is involved while changing over from the bottom position to the upward movement. Once again, when your form starts to get sloppy, STOP! Either reduce the weight or take a rest in preparation for the next set.

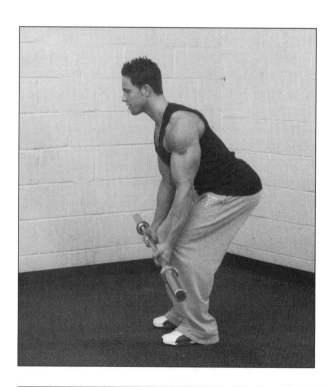 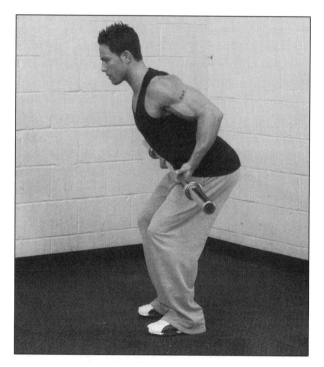

Mind Over Muscle Re-MIND-er:

Imagine there are steel cables and one end is attached to your elbows. The other end is connected to an electric winch on the ceiling above you. That winch just keeps pulling and pulling and your elbows are drawn up and up until that bar nearly touches your chest. Keep these images strong and active in your mind during the execution of the exercise. It might feel awkward at first, but once you get that image locked in your head you'll be very surprised at how well they work! (And how hard it is to get rid of the image!)

T-Bar Row

PRIMARY TARGET MUSCLES: Mid Back, Latissimus Dorsi

NOTES: T-bar rows hit the back muscles slightly differently than a barbell row, much like a close grip pull-up attacks the lats differently than a wide-grip pull-up. You can use a T-bar anchor or a wall corner for this exercise as well.

EXECUTION AND FORM

Step 1: Load the seated T-bar row machine with a moderate amount of weight.

Step 2: Straddle the machine with your feet about shoulder width apart. Make sure your knees are pointing directly in front of you and are slightly bent throughout the movement.

Step 3: Bend over at the hips, making sure that your lower back is not slumped over. To make sure of this, squeeze or contract your abdominal and glute muscles while slightly arching your lower back. Do not bend over all the way as this can injure the lower back. Your back should be parallel to the floor or slightly higher. But if you stand too upright, this positioning will not sufficiently activate the back muscles. You must be bent over to a degree where the elbows will naturally remain close to the body. At the same time, the back of the arms (triceps) follow a row-like movement, directly toward the ceiling.

Step 4: Pick up the T-bar using either a palms-down or a palms-up type of grip. The palms-down grip is recommended for beginners, as with this grip the biceps are less involved. Advanced exercisers can use a palms-up grip, which will stress the lats more directly. As you pick up the bar, think about which muscles you are about to exercise. The lats are located on the outermost side of the back and are your focus point.

Step 5: Let the bar hang down. Keep the elbows slightly wider than shoulder width.

Step 6: Stick out your chest while slightly squeezing your shoulder blades together. This will position and keep your body in the proper alignment throughout the movement. Holding these alignment positions throughout the exercise will help make sure that stimulation remains in the back muscles.

Step 7: Contract your upper back muscles, and begin rowing the elbows up toward the ceiling, allowing the back of the arms (triceps) to lead the motion.

Step 8: Drive the elbows and back of the arms upward until the weight is touching your chest or you've fully contracted the back muscles. Imagine that there is an egg in the middle of your back. Your objective for each repetition, when the bar is being pulled to your belly, is to crack the egg with your back muscles.

Step 9: Keep your head up and looking straight ahead throughout the movement. This will help you keep your balance and make it easier to maintain the described position.

Step 10: Try to squeeze the muscles at the top of the movement, and learn to isolate those specific muscles. When you apply this technique to an exercise, you are actually optimizing your training sessions through the increased muscle recruitment.

Step 11: Begin the descent with a slow and controlled movement. As you

T-Bar Row

SECONDARY TARGET MUSCLES: Lower Back, Rear Deltoids, Biceps

reach the bottom, slowly and smoothly begin the movement upward again without resting. Make sure that no momentum is involved while changing over from the bottom position to the upward movement. Once again, when your form starts to get sloppy, STOP! Either reduce the weight or take a rest in preparation for the next set.

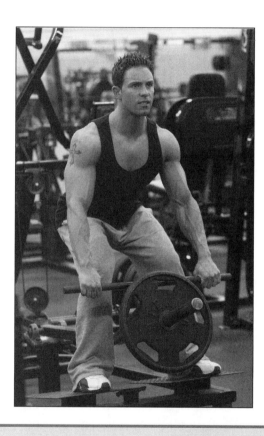 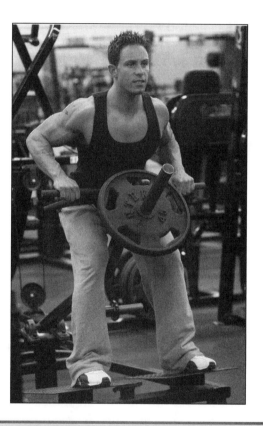

Mind Over Muscle Re-MIND-er:

Increase your ability to concentrate on an exercise by challenging yourself. Every so often, try lifting heavier weights than you normally do. Occasionally do more reps than your workout calls for, or rest less between sets. Any time you challenge yourself physically you also stimulate mental awareness, which will pay off in a more effective workout. You'll also stimulate your muscles further, which leads to more growth. Don't be afraid to come out of your comfort zone by challenging yourself. Just make sure that you are not biting off more than you can chew, as you want to avoid any chance of injury.

T-Bar Machine Row

PRIMARY TARGET MUSCLES: **Mid Back, Latissimus Dorsi**

NOTES: This exercise allows you to handle much greater weights without the strain on the lower back. It is highly recommended for trainees with lower back problems.

EXECUTION AND FORM

Step 1: Load the T-bar machine with a moderate weight, then sit down and place your chest or abdomen on the support pad.

Step 2: Reach over the support pad with your arms and grasp the handles using either a palms-down or a palms-up type of grip. The palms-down grip is recommended for beginners, because with this grip the biceps are less involved. Advanced exercisers can use a palms-up grip, which will stress the lats more directly. As you grip the handles, think about what muscles you are about to exercise. The lats are located on the outermost side of the back and are your focus point.

Step 3: Let the T-bar hang from your arms, but not so far that it bottoms out. Keep the elbows slightly wider than shoulder width.

Step 4: Stick out your chest while slightly squeezing your shoulder blades together. This will position and keep your body in the proper alignment throughout the movement. Holding these alignment positions throughout the exercise will help make sure that stimulation remains in the back muscles.

Step 5: Contract your upper back muscles, and begin rowing the elbows up toward the ceiling, allowing the back of the arms (triceps) to lead the motion.

Step 6: Drive the elbows and back of the arms upward until the weight is touching your chest or you've fully contracted the back muscles. Imagine that there is an egg in the middle of your back. Your objective for each repetition, when the bar is being pulled to your belly, is to crack the egg with your back muscles.

Step 7: Keep your head up and looking straight ahead throughout the movement. This will help you keep your balance and make it easier to maintain the described position.

Step 8: Try to squeeze the muscles at the top of the movement, and learn to isolate those specific muscles. When you apply this technique to an exercise, you are actually optimizing your training sessions through the increased muscle recruitment.

Step 9: Begin the descent with a slow and controlled movement. As you reach the bottom, slowly and smoothly begin the movement upward again without resting. Make sure that no momentum is involved while changing over from the bottom position to the upward movement. Once again, when your form starts to get sloppy, STOP! Either reduce the weight or take a rest in preparation for the next set.

T-Bar Machine Row

SECONDARY TARGET MUSCLES: **Lower Back, Rear Deltoids, Biceps**

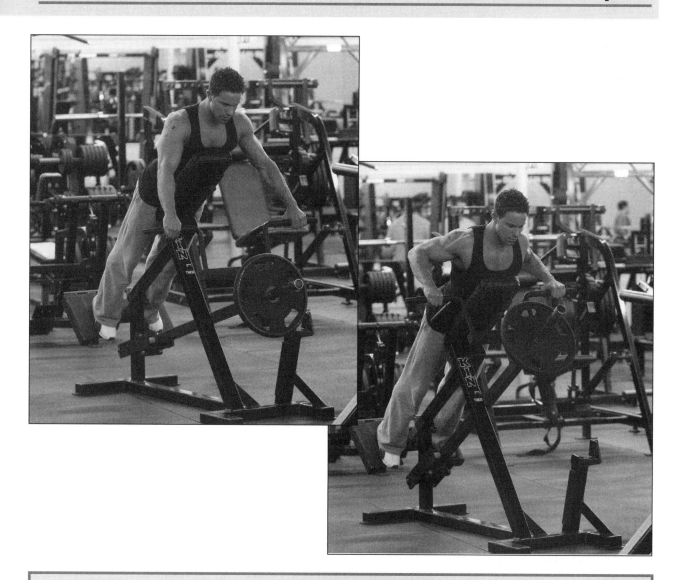

Mind Over Muscle Re-MIND-er:

Be careful not to involve your lower back during rowing motions. Doing so can promote injury. Instead of thinking that you are pulling on the bar, think that you are squeezing your shoulder blades together (and cracking that darn egg!!!). This will keep your focus on the upper and mid back muscles, where it belongs.

97

Towel Row

PRIMARY TARGET MUSCLES: **Mid Back, Latissimus Dorsi**

NOTES: When you are traveling or don't have access to weights and machines, you can replace barbell, T-bar, or T-bar Machine Rows with Towel Rows. Towel rows have the same movement as other rows, but instead of pulling a weight toward you, you're going to pull your body toward an object.

EXECUTION AND FORM

Step 1: Use a large, thick hotel towel or a length of rope for this exercise.

Step 2: Loop the middle of your towel or rope around a pole or other stationary object and hold onto one end in each hand.

Step 3: Sit on the floor in front of the pole with your toes touching the door and your knees bent at a 90-degree angle. Tense your leg muscles so that your knees and hips remain bent at approximately the same angle through the whole exercise.

Step 4: Now pull your bodyweight off the floor using your lats and arms. If this is too easy for you, you can do one arm at a time by grabbing both ends of the towel in the same hand. You'll likely need to rotate your torso toward the working hand to maintain your balance.

Step 5: If the two-hand method is too difficult, you can sit on the floor and loop the towel around one or both feet. Straighten your leg(s) and use a rowing motion to pull your foot toward you while actively resisting with your leg muscles.

Towel Row

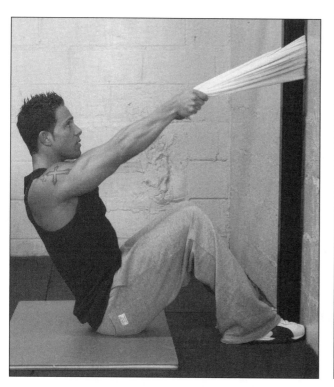

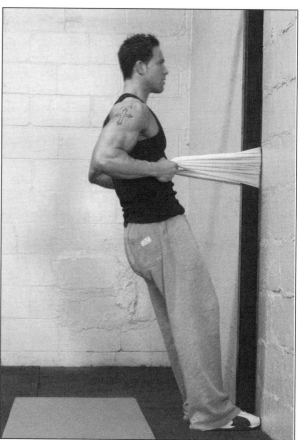

Mind Over Muscle Re-MIND-er:

Using the Full Body Tension technique will help you to maintain your posture throughout the exercise, and increase the number of reps you are able to do.

One-Arm Dumbbell Row

PRIMARY TARGET MUSCLES: **Upper Back**

NOTES: The one-arm dumbbell row allows you to concentrate on one side of the back at a time, which is good for preventing or correcting imbalances between the two sides. The one-arm row also lets you use a much heavier dumbbell without putting extra strain on your back.

EXECUTION AND FORM

Step 1: Find a flat bench and set a dumbbell at the right side of it. Position your right foot on the floor while positioning your left knee on the bench. Your left hand should be positioned slightly in front of your body on the bench. Lean slightly into your left hand to help support your body weight. Pick up the dumbbell with your right hand using a neutral grip, with palms facing your body and thumbs pointing forward. Remember to support your body weight with your left hand. If you have back problems or feel unstable with this particular foot stance, bring your right foot out to make your stance wider. Also, instead of pulling the dumbbell up across your thigh, pull it up in between your body and leg. This slight modification will make sure your back is safe, especially for heavier lifting.

Step 2: With your arm hanging straight, lift the dumbbell off the floor until your back is flat and parallel to the floor. Look straight ahead to help maintain balance and form. Do not look down or up during the exercise.

Step 3: Think about the muscles you are about to exercise: the latissimus dorsi, or "lats." Contract them isometrically before beginning the lift.

Step 4: Slightly lift the shoulder blade, making sure that it maintains a level position. Begin rowing the elbow up toward the ceiling, allowing the back of the arm (triceps) to lead the motion. Row the elbow and back of the arm up toward the ceiling. Row as far as you can until the back of the arm and elbow reach the level of the torso. Make sure that you are fully contracting the back muscles. Try to reach over with your working shoulder blade and touch the non-working shoulder blade.

Step 5: Squeeze and hold that position, focusing on an intense contraction of the back muscles. Begin your descent with a slow and controlled movement.

Step 6: As you reach the bottom, slowly and smoothly begin the movement upward again without resting. Make sure that no momentum is involved when changing over from the bottom position back to the upward movement. When your form starts to get sloppy, STOP! Either reduce the weight, or take a rest in preparation for the next set.

One-Arm Dumbbell Row

SECONDARY TARGET MUSCLES: Biceps

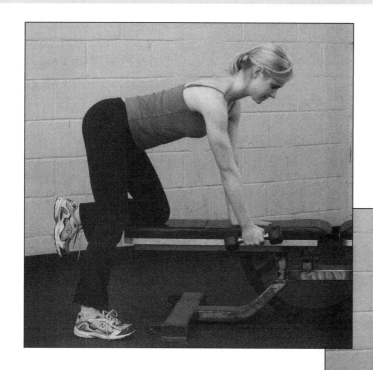

Mind Over Muscle Re-MIND-er:

Take your mind off your biceps by driving up with your elbows instead of pulling with your arms. Just let your forearms be huge, dangling hooks. As you drive the elbows up, make sure that resistance is kept on the upper back muscles—think about pulling your upper arms up toward the ceiling.

Two-Arm Dumbbell Row

PRIMARY TARGET MUSCLES: Upper Back

NOTES: Although we recommend the pronated grip in this exercise, it can also be done with a neutral grip or supinated grip. As you advance in this program, try the other two grips from time to time as they will attack your lats and biceps from different angles and help develop them completely.

EXECUTION AND FORM

Step 1: Place two dumbbells on the floor in front of your feet. With knees slightly bent, bend over at the hips and grasp one in each hand using a pronated grip, with palms facing behind you and thumbs pointing toward your body.

Step 2: With your arms hanging straight, lift the dumbbells off the floor until your back is parallel to the floor. The back should be flat as you lean over from the hips and you should be looking straight ahead to help maintain balance and form. Do not look down or up during the exercise.

Step 3: Pause to consciously think about the muscles you are about to exercise: the latissimus dorsi, or "lats."

Step 4: Slightly lift the shoulder blades, making sure they maintain a level position. Begin rowing the elbows up toward the ceiling, allowing the back of the arms (triceps) to lead the motion. Row as far back as you can until the back of the arm and elbow reach the level of the torso. Make sure that you are fully contracting the back muscles. If it helps, imagine that there is an egg in the middle of your mid-back. Your objective, when the weight is being rowed, is to squeeze the back muscles and crack the egg with your back muscles.

Step 5: Squeeze and hold that position, focusing on an intense contraction of the back muscles. Begin your descent with a slow and controlled movement.

Step 6: As you reach the bottom, slowly and smoothly begin the movement upward again without resting. Make sure that no momentum is involved when changing over from the bottom position back to the upward movement. When your form starts to get sloppy, STOP! Either reduce the weight, or take a rest in preparation for the next set.

Two-Arm Dumbbell Row

SECONDARY TARGET MUSCLES: **Biceps**

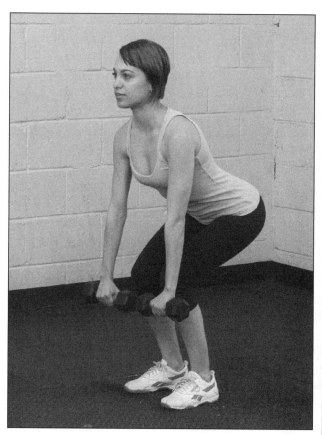

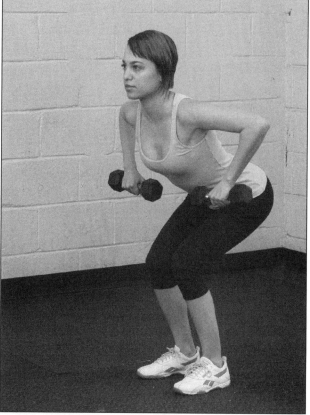

Mind Over Muscle Re-MIND-er:

Get your mind into your muscles and mentally picture the individual muscle fibers being recruited and activating even as you are contracting. Imagine that the harder the exercise becomes, the more your muscles are developing and the more they can handle. Always use strong, positive images when visualizing your muscle fibers, such as wire, rope, or steel cables, and your workout will benefit from this mindfulness.

Seated Machine Row

PRIMARY TARGET MUSCLES: Mid Back, Lower Lats

NOTES: Rowing exercises simulate rowing a boat to target the upper and middle back muscles. Some rowing machines allow you to push your elbows back instead of pulling them, which takes the biceps out of the equation so you can focus more on the back muscles. Seated rows should be done with two hands, and with a supinated, pronated or neutral grip, depending on the kinds of handles available. We recommend either the neutral or pronated grips. Choose a neutral grip to target muscles in the mid back, and a pronated grip to hit the lats more, depending on which muscles you feel need more development.

EXECUTION AND FORM

Step 1: Sit in the machine's chair. If you have a choice of handles, attach the appropriate handle for the grip you plan to use.

Step 2: Brace your feet against the plate provided with your knees slightly bent. Grip the handles with straight arms and bring your torso to an upright position.

Step 3: Focus your attention on your lats. With the weight pulling your arms out in front of you, the mus-cles you feel being stretched under your arms are your lats. Begin to flex your lats.

Step 4: You will find that tensing your legs and lower back while contract-ing your glutes keeps your body in the correct posture and position dur-ing this exercise. It's important that you not sway forward and back dur-ing the pulling motion as this risks injuring the lower back muscles.

Step 5: When you can feel and flex your lats, squeeze the grip with your hands and begin pulling with your lats. Pull the handle toward your abdomen and as your elbows move past your body squeeze your shoul-der blades together as if you're squeezing a ball between them.

Step 6: Slowly return to the starting position. Remember to resist the weight as your arms extend.

Seated Machine Row

SECONDARY TARGET MUSCLES: **Lower Back, Biceps**

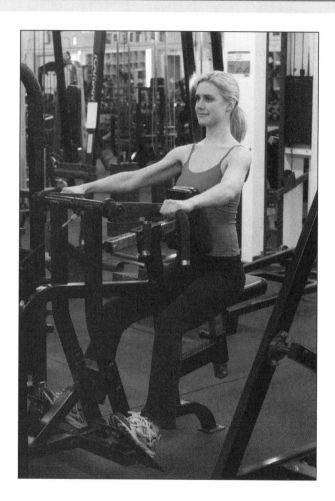

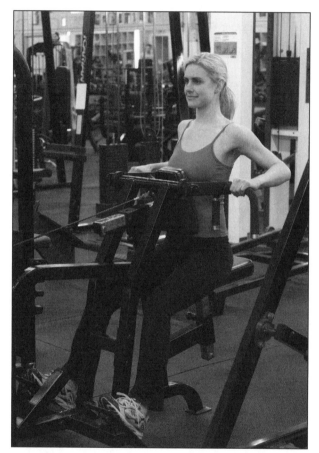

Mind Over Muscle Re-MIND-er:

Instead of thinking about heaving weights in a gym, imagine you are actually rescuing a loved one who's drowning in the middle of a lake. You're rowing a boat to reach them and bring them back to safety. It's your spouse, child, parent, girlfriend/ boyfriend, sister, brother or whoever is dearest to you—and if you quit now, they'll drown.

Plate-Loaded One-Arm Row

PRIMARY TARGET MUSCLES: Mid Back, Lower Lats

NOTES: A seated one-arm row allows you to prevent or correct muscle imbalances in the upper back. Some rowing machines allow you to push your elbows back instead of pulling them, which takes the biceps out of the equation so you can focus more on the back muscles.

EXECUTION AND FORM

Step 1: Sit in the machine's chair. Brace your feet against the plate provided with your knees slightly bent. Grip the handle with a neutral, or vertical, grip and with a straight arm bring your torso to an upright position. With your non-working hand, grab onto a stationary handle or other support to provide balance.

Step 2: Focus your attention on your lats. With the weight pulling your arm out in front of you, the muscles you feel being stretched under your shoulders are your lats. Flex the lats on the side you're working.

Step 3: You will find that tensing your legs and lower back while contracting your glutes keeps your body in the correct posture and position during this exercise. It's important that you not sway forward and back during the pulling motion as this risks injuring the lower back muscles.

Step 4: When you can feel and flex your lats, squeeze the grip with your hands and begin pulling with your lats. Pull the handle toward your abdomen and as your elbows move past your body squeeze your shoulder blades together, rotating your working shoulder blade across your back to try and touch the opposite shoulder blade.

Step 5: Hold the contraction and slowly return to the starting position. Remember to resist the weight as your arms extend.

Plate-Loaded One-Arm Row

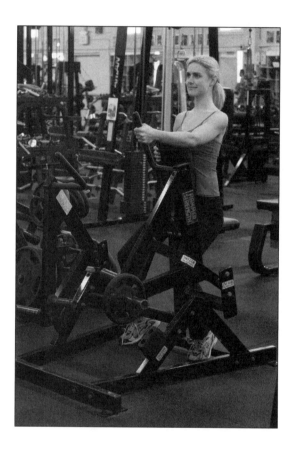
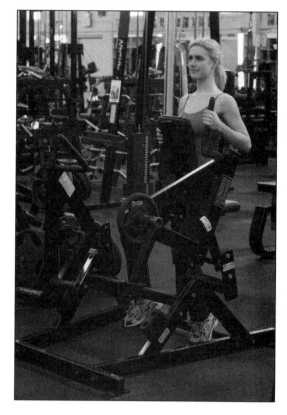

Mind Over Muscle Re-MIND-er:

The muscles involved in this exercise can be difficult to isolate in your mind. You'll tend to think of your arm first. But ignore the arm; it's the muscles behind your shoulder blade that you are trying to work. Focus on your shoulder blade and mentally draw it back and across your back to the opposite side. If it helps, picture your shoulder blades as containing wings, and flap them!

Low Pulley Row

PRIMARY TARGET MUSCLES: **Mid Back, Lower Lats**

NOTES: Like the machine rows, seated row pulley rows allow you to work the upper back without straining the lower back by bending over. If you don't have a machine available, using pulleys is a good alternative to the machine row.

EXECUTION AND FORM

Step 1: Sit on the floor in front of the low pulley. If you have a choice of handles, attach a handle that allows you to use a neutral grip.

Step 2: Brace your feet against the plate provided, or against two 45-pound plates set flat on the floor against the pulley frame. You should have a foot on either side of the pulley cable and your knees should be slightly bent.

Step 3: Grip the handlebar and with straight arms bring your torso to an upright position.

Step 4: Focus your attention on your lats. With the weight pulling your arms out in front of you, the muscles you feel being stretched beneath your shoulder are your lats. Begin to flex your lats.

Step 5: You will find that tensing your legs and lower back while contracting your glutes keeps your body in the correct posture and position during this exercise. It's important that you not sway forward and back during the pulling motion as this risks injuring the lower back muscles.

Step 6: When you can feel and flex your lats, squeeze the grip with your hands and begin pulling with your lats. Pull the handlebar toward your abdomen and as your elbows come past your body squeeze your shoulder blades together as if you're squeezing a ball between them.

Step 7: Hold the contraction and slowly return to the starting position. Make sure you resist the weight on the way back while continuing to concentrate on the contraction of your lats.

Low Pulley Row

SECONDARY TARGET MUSCLES: **Lower Back, Biceps**

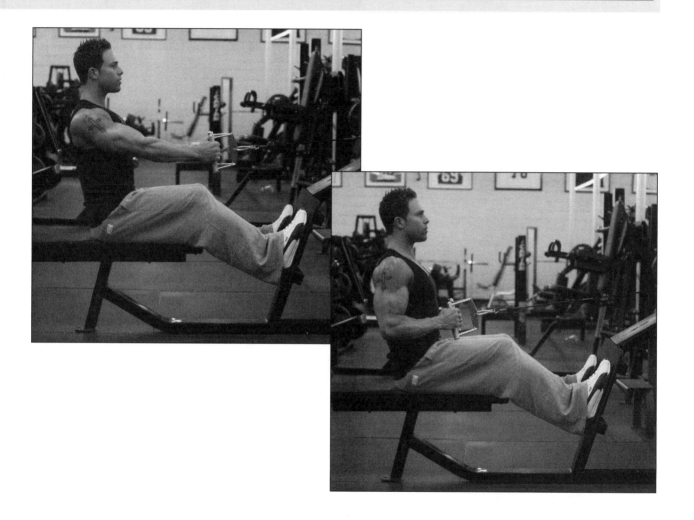

Mind Over Muscle Re-MIND-er:

Although seated rowing exercises simulate rowing a boat, be careful not to involve your lower back. Doing so promotes injury. Instead of thinking that you are pulling on the bar, think that you are squeezing your shoulder blades together (as if cracking an egg between them). This will keep your focus on the upper back muscles where it should be. As you pull your arms back, simultaneously stick your chest out. This movement is similar to the Screw Tension Technique, in that you are gaining leverage through opposition.

Standing High Pulley V-Bar Row

PRIMARY TARGET MUSCLES: Mid Back, Lower Lats

NOTES: This exercise hits your back muscles from a different angle than bent over rows or seated low-pulley rows, giving your back muscles an appearance of completeness.

EXECUTION AND FORM

Step 1: Find a station where you can bring the cable attachment higher than you are or go to a lat pulldown station. Attach a V-bar to the hook and take your grip on the bar.

Step 2: Select a weight and position your body as follows: Feet should be hip width apart, knees slightly bent, abs tight, chest out, and shoulders back and relaxed downward.

Step 3: With arms fully extended, lean back. Be sure to keep your chest out and shoulders back and down.

Step 4: Contract your back muscles isometrically and draw your concentration into those muscles. Tighten your abs and stabilize your body position as you begin to pull the bar towards your chest. Throughout the movement, try to keep your elbows a bit tighter to your body. If the elbows float away, you will not be isolating your back muscles.

Step 5: Do your best to avoid using momentum, as it will greatly impact your ability to isolate those back muscles.

Step 6: As you reach the point where the bar is touching your chest, contract the back muscles as hard as possible, hold, and slowly come back to the starting, fully extended position. Without resting, begin pulling the bar back toward your chest, for the desired number of repetitions.

Standing High Pulley V-Bar Row

SECONDARY TARGET MUSCLES: Lower Back, Biceps

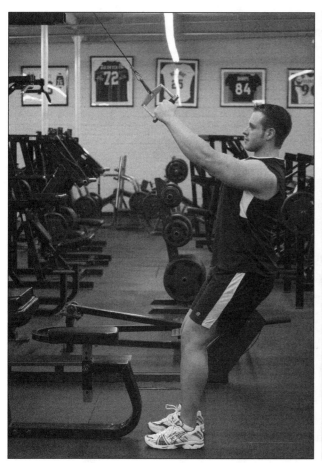 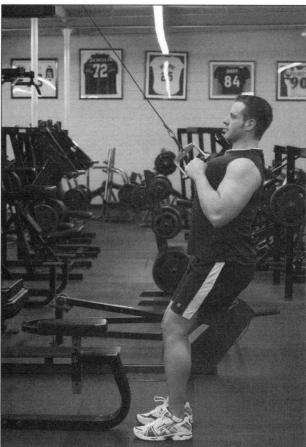

Mind Over Muscle Re-MIND-er:

Music is a great tool to help you stay focused while training. If you train in a public gym and they don't play uplifting and good beat/tempo music, bring your own. It doesn't matter what genre of music you play, but it is important that the beat of the song be a solid cadence. Something too slow or too quick can be disruptive to your training. Listen to a number of songs at home and try to find music that fits the Two-Step Rep cadence: "1-up- 1-hold- 1-down" and make a compilation of songs you like with that tempo.

Wide Grip Pullup

PRIMARY TARGET MUSCLES: Latissimus Dorsi

NOTES: The wide-grip pull-up is the champion of upper back exercises and will pack a lot of size onto your lats. If you cannot pull your own body weight up, try a Gravitron machine, which assists you in pulling your body weight. If Gravitrons are not available to you, then try one of these:
  • Have someone provide assistance by holding your legs;
  • Put your feet on a chair in front of or behind you and assist the pull with your legs;
  • Use the pulldown machines until you're strong enough for pullups.

EXECUTION AND FORM

Step 1: Grab onto an overhead bar or pulldown bar with an overhand grip, placing your hands about 1 ½ times your shoulder width apart. Different hand spacing will focus on different muscles. The grip I suggest reduces biceps use to focus more on stimulating the back muscles.

Step 2: Let your body hang while bending your knees to get your feet off the floor and crossing your ankles. Contract your abdominal section, which helps to sustain your postural alignment throughout the movement.

Step 3: Stick your chest out while pressing your shoulders downward, which will help isolate the intended musculature of the back. Focus on your lats and begin to contract them.

Step 4: Keeping your elbows as wide as you can, begin pulling your chest toward the bar. Throughout the movement keep your head and eyes looking up. Knowing that you must reach your target position at the top adds that extra push. Squeezing the bar with your hands will help you keep the tension you need on your lats to get you to the top.

Step 5: When you reach the top, which is when you can no longer move upward while maintaining the proper alignment, consciously focus on squeezing and contracting the back muscles as hard as you can. Try to hold that contraction to help isolate the back muscles.

Step 6: As you begin your descent, slowly lower your body while mentally focusing on the back muscles being activated. When you feel yourself fatiguing or losing control on the way down, try to pull back up. You'll notice that as you get tired, even your best attempt to pull yourself back up will not stop your descent. This technique will add some additional intensity and overall stimulation of the back muscles.

Step 7: For a full range of motion, let your arms straighten completely at the bottom of the movement. Most people only come down two-thirds of the way and leave out perhaps the most important portion of the exercise—the fully stretched position. Next, slowly and smoothly begin the transition upward once again without using any momentum.

Wide Grip Pullup

SECONDARY TARGET MUSCLES: **Biceps, Serratus**

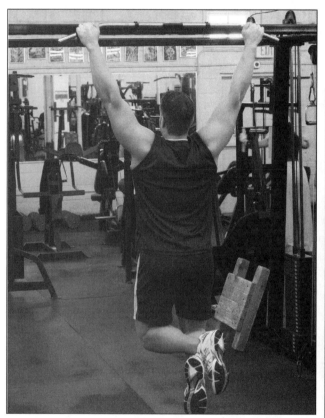 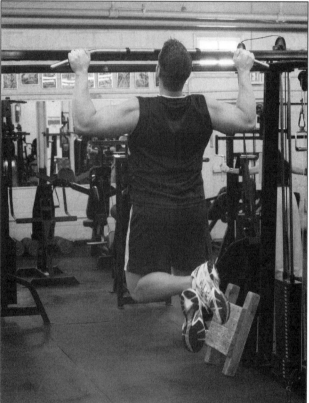

Mind Over Muscle Re-MIND-er:

To focus your mind on the back muscles, think about your shoulder blades and that they are leveraging your arms to push yourself up—do not think "pull!" If you think "pull," you will engage more of your biceps and your lats may not get the full benefit of the exercise. Remind yourself to not use momentum to pull up. Keep your chest out and head looking up. The Flushing technique is great for getting through those sticking points.

Narrow Grip V-Bar Pullup

PRIMARY TARGET MUSCLES: Latissimus Dorsi

NOTES: Using a V-bar or close-grip bar for pullups hits the lats in a slightly different way, and brings the serratus muscles more into play. Again, if you can't do enough pullups with your body weight, use one of the alternatives listed under Wide Grip Pullups.

EXECUTION AND FORM

Step 1: With the V-bar placed over a chinning bar, grab the handles with your palms facing each other.

Step 2: Let your body hang while bending your knees and crossing your feet. Contract your abdominal section, which helps to sustain your postural alignment throughout the movement.

Step 3: Keep your elbows as wide as you can as you begin pulling your chest toward the bar. Lean your head backward slightly so that your chest can touch the V-bar (or almost touch it). You may also have to duck your head to one side to avoid hitting it on the chinning bar. If you do,

alternate sides with every rep to avoid muscle imbalances.

Step 4: When you reach the top, which will be when you can no longer move upward while maintaining the proper alignment, consciously focus on squeezing and contracting the back muscles as hard as you can.

Step 5: As you begin your descent, slowly lower your body while mentally focusing on the back muscles being activated. When you feel yourself fatiguing or losing control on the way down, try to pull back up. You'll notice that as you get tired, even your best attempt to pull

yourself back up will not stop your descent. This technique will add some additional intensity and overall stimulation of the back muscles.

Step 6: For a full range of motion, let your arms straighten completely at the bottom of the movement. Most people only come down two-thirds of the way and leave out perhaps the most important portion of the exercise—the fully stretched position. Next, slowly and smoothly, begin the transition upward once again without using any momentum.

Narrow Grip V-Bar Pullup

SECONDARY TARGET MUSCLES: **Biceps, Serratus**

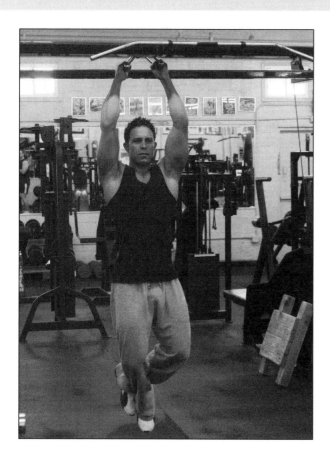

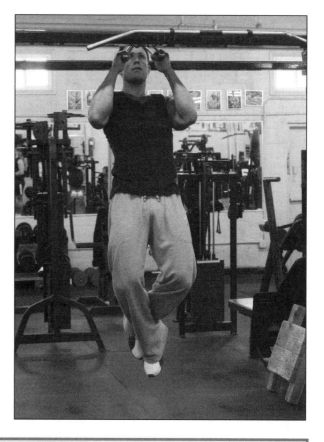

Mind Over Muscle Re-MIND-er:

Having trouble with the last rep in your set? Imagine there's an invisible person spotting you and he's there to help you pull those last grueling inches to the bar. They can lift as hard as you need them to, and unlike "real" spotters are always there when you need them!

Wide Grip Pulldown

PRIMARY TARGET MUSCLES: **Latissimus Dorsi**

NOTES: This exercise is very similar to the wide grip pullup in how it impacts the lats. However, where pullup repetitions are limited by your body weight, you can continue to do more pulldown repetitions by lowering the weight. Pulldowns are great if you can't pull up your body weight yet or after you've done as many pullups as you can.

EXECUTION AND FORM

Step 1: Seated at a pulldown machine, grab the pulldown bar with an overhand grip with your hands about 1 ½ times your shoulder width apart. If the bar has angled hand grips, use those. Different hand spacing will focus on different muscles. The grip I suggest reduces biceps use to focus more on stimulating the back muscles.

Step 2: Put your knees under the support pad provided. This will keep you from pulling yourself off the seat when the weight gets heavy.

Step 3: Stick your chest out and focus on your lats. Contract them isometrically.

Step 4: Keep your elbows as wide as you can, and begin pulling the bar toward your chest. Throughout the movement keep your head and eyes looking up.

Step 5: When you reach the full contraction, consciously focus on squeezing and contracting the back muscles as hard as you can. Hold that contraction to isolate the back muscles.

Step 6: Slowly return your arms to the starting position while resisting the weight. At the starting position, start your next rep without stopping, jerking or using momentum. Instead, make the transition slow and fluid.

Wide Grip Pulldown

SECONDARY TARGET MUSCLES: **Biceps, Serratus**

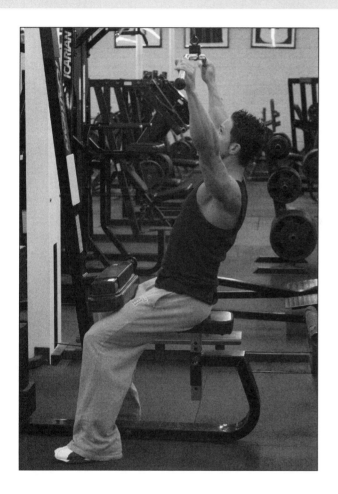
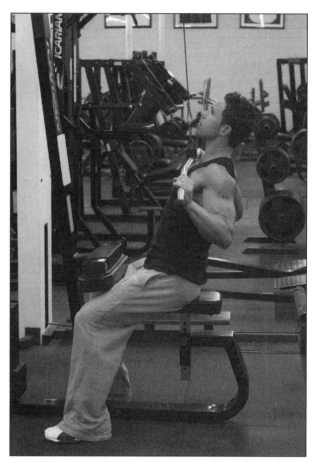

Mind Over Muscle Re-MIND-er:

Back muscles can be difficult to visualize because unlike our biceps or abs we never see them. Instead, watch the backs of other lifters to see how their muscles contract. Then look at yours in a mirror and get them to contract in the same way. Pay attention to what the movement feels like so you can duplicate it during your workout, and always keep the mental image in mind as you continue to exercise. The Flushing technique is great for getting stronger here too.

High Pulley V-Bar Pulldown

PRIMARY TARGET MUSCLES: **Latissimus Dorsi**

NOTES: This exercise is very similar to the V-bar pullup in how it impacts the lats. However, where pullup repetitions are limited by your body weight, you can continue to do more pulldown repetitions by lowering the weight. Pulldowns are great if you can't pull up your body weight yet or after you've done as many pullups as you can.

EXECUTION AND FORM

Step 1: Seated at a pulldown machine with a V-bar attached, grab the handles of the V-bar with your palms facing each other.

Step 2: Put your knees under the support pad provided. This will keep you from pulling yourself off the seat when the weight gets heavy.

Step 3: Contract the lats isometrically. Concentrate on the contraction throughout the exercise.

Step 4: Keeping your elbows as wide as you can, begin pulling the V-bar toward your chest. Lean your head backward slightly so that you can touch the V-bar to your chest (or almost touch it).

Step 5: When you reach the full contraction, consciously focus on squeezing and contracting the back muscles as hard as you can. Hold that contraction to isolate the back muscles.

Step 6: Slowly return your arms to the starting position while resisting the weight. At the starting position start your next rep without stopping, jerking or using momentum. Make the transition slow and fluid instead.

High Pulley V-Bar Pulldown

SECONDARY TARGET MUSCLES: **Biceps, Serratus**

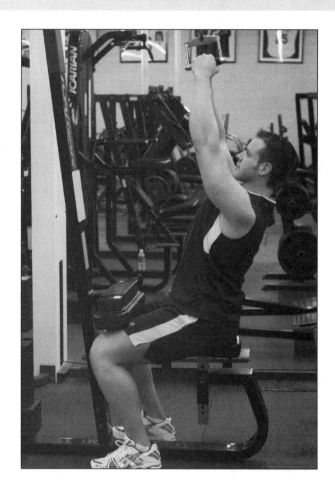

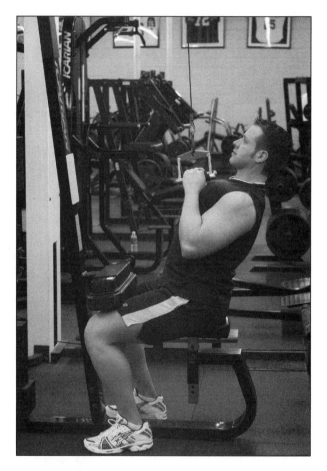

Mind Over Muscle Re-MIND-er:

Before you begin ANY exercise, take a moment or two to picture yourself performing the upcoming exercise successfully and correctly. Once you've got that perfect picture in your head, rewind the tape and play it again several times. Once you're ready to actually begin that exercise, your body will do it's best to imitate what you've imagined and make the exercise much more effective.

Close Reverse Grip Pulldown

PRIMARY TARGET MUSCLES: Latissimus Dorsi

NOTES: The close reverse grip pulldown attacks the lats from yet another angle, again bringing the serratus into play. The biceps have more of a role in this pulldown, but it gives the lats a full stretch that they don't get in other pulldown exercises. Reduce the role of the biceps by pulling your elbows back instead of your hands.

EXECUTION AND FORM

Step 1: Seated at a pulldown machine, grab the pulldown bar with a supinated or underhand grip, with your palms facing you and your hands 4 to 6 inches apart.

Step 2: Put your knees under the support pad provided. This will keep you from pulling yourself off the seat when the weight gets heavy.

Step 3: Contract the lats isometrically.

Step 4: Keep your elbows as wide as you can and begin pulling the bar toward your sternum. Throughout the movement keep your head and eyes looking up.

Step 5: When you reach the full contraction, consciously focus on squeezing and contracting the back muscles as hard as you can. Hold that contraction to isolate the back muscles.

Step 6: Slowly return your arms to the starting position while resisting the weight. At the starting position start your next rep without stopping, without jerking, and without using momentum. Make the transition slow and fluid.

Close Reverse Grip Pulldown

SECONDARY TARGET MUSCLES: **Biceps, Serratus**

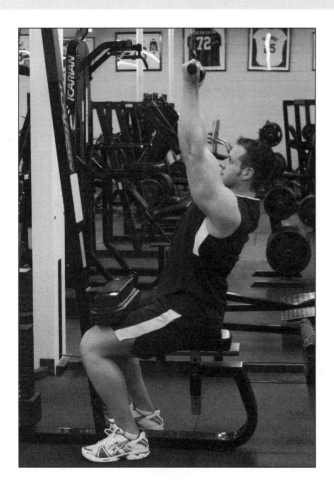
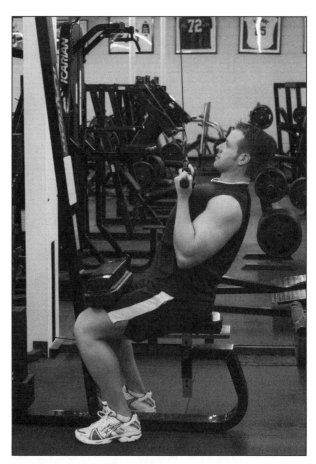

Mind Over Muscle Re-MIND-er:

It's difficult to perform well if you're feeling tense or agitated. Deep breathing is a simple but extremely effective way to relax in a short amount of time. Take a moment and find a place to sit down and close your eyes. Inhale deeply (through your nose) into your diaphragm (stomach), and then into your chest. Take 5 to 10 seconds to complete the inhale. Exhale slowly (out through your mouth). Start by emptying your chest and then your diaphragm, taking equal time or longer to exhale as you did to inhale. As the breath leaves your body, imagine all the anxiety and tension exiting your body through your head and into the atmosphere. A good 10 breaths and you should be ready for that workout.

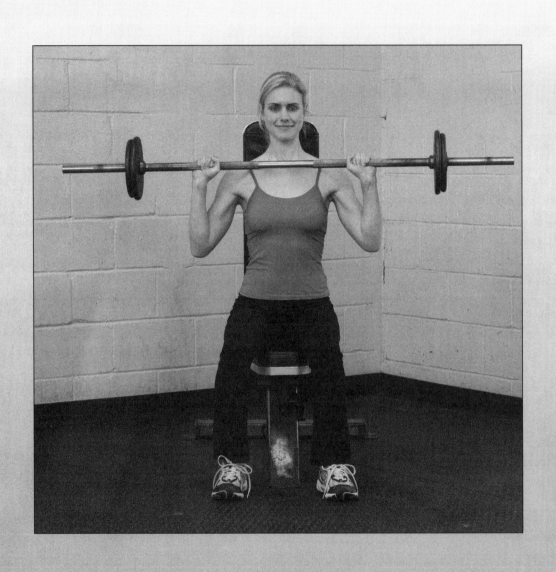

Chapter 7:

Shoulder and Arm Exercises

Shoulders

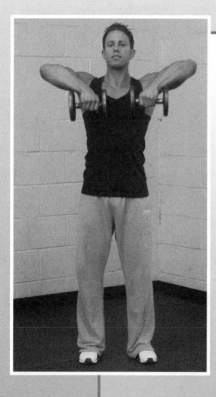

- E-Z Bar Upright Row

- Dumbbell Upright Row

- Dumbbell Shrug

- Smith Machine Shrug

- Barbell Shoulder Press

- Dumbbell Shoulder Press

- Handstand Press

- Dumbbell Lateral Raise

- Bent-Over Lateral Raise

- Rear Deltoid Machine

- Isometric Lateral Raise

E-Z Bar Upright Row

PRIMARY TARGET MUSCLES: Deltoids, Trapezius

NOTES: The rotator cuff muscles of the shoulder are extremely delicate and are prone to injuries that occur because of poor form and excessive weight. So it's imperative that you use a weight you can handle and use perfect form and technique with no momentum at all. I recommend that you practice the exercise using an E-Z Curl bar at first, if possible, which is easier on the wrists and shoulders than a straight barbell.

EXECUTION AND FORM

Step 1: Choose a weight for the E-Z bar that is easy enough so that you can focus on your form. Once you have mastered the correct form, it will become second nature and you will find it easy to move up in weight, thereby being able to fully stimulate the shoulder muscles.

Step 2: Grasp the bar using a shoulder width or slightly narrower grip. Stand with your feet shoulder width apart and point them straight ahead. Keep your knees slightly bent at all times during the movement to take stress off the lower back region. Also, keep the knees pointing straight ahead.

Step 3: Contract the abdominal muscles slightly to help keep your postural alignment. Keep your back straight, body still, and your head level and looking straight ahead as you do the exercise.

Step 4: Relax the musculature of your chest and back. Close your eyes and once again visualize yourself actually doing the movement while focusing on the shoulder and trapezius muscles.

Step 5: Hold the bar across your thighs and keep your palms facing toward your body. Focus on the muscles of the shoulder, including the trapezius muscles, which run across your upper back. Although you will be pulling the weight up with your hands, you must let the elbows lead the motion, keeping them high as you pull up.

Step 6: Begin pulling the bar up slowly, concentrating on feeling the stimulation of the focused muscles. Lead with your elbows, and lift the bar to a point where it comes close to your chin. The most important thing to do at this position of the exercise is to consciously focus on and physically contract the muscles of the trapezius. Hold the contraction here. Make sure not to hold the bar too close to your body, as this can injure the rotator cuff muscles. Hold the bar about 6 inches away from your body as you pull the bar upward.

Step 7: Slowly lower the bar while maintaining the same exact form and posture you did when pulling up. When you reach the bottom position, slowly begin pulling the bar back to the top position of the exercise using a controlled, fluid motion. Make sure that you do not jerk or use momentum to lift the bar at any time during this exercise.

E-Z Bar Upright Row

SECONDARY TARGET MUSCLES: **Biceps**

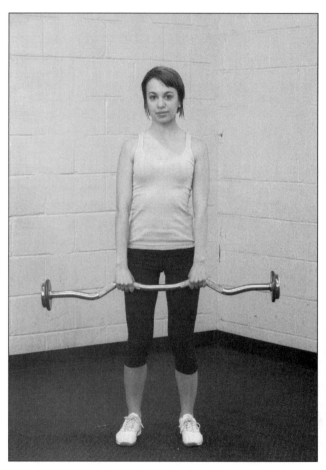
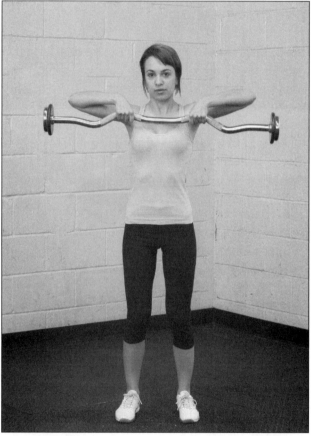

Mind Over Muscle Re-MIND-er:

This exercise requires full concentration and focus to stay tight and straight. The Full Body Tension technique is ideal for upright rows, because it contracts every muscle in your body, which keeps it locked in alignment.

Dumbbell Upright Row

PRIMARY TARGET MUSCLES: Deltoids, Trapezius

NOTES: The rotator cuff muscles of the shoulder are extremely delicate and are prone to injuries that occur because of poor form and excessive weight. So it's imperative that you use a weight you can handle and use perfect form and technique with no momentum at all.

EXECUTION AND FORM

Step 1: Choose a weight that is easy enough so that you can focus on your form. Once you have mastered the correct form, it will become second nature and you will find it easy to move up in weight, thereby being able to fully stimulate the shoulder muscles.

Step 2: Stand with the dumbbells in a pronated grip so that your hands are directly in front of your thighs. Place your feet shoulder width apart and point them straight ahead. Keep your knees slightly bent at all times during the movement to take stress off the lower back region. Also, keep the knees pointing straight ahead.

Step 3: Contract the abdominal muscles slightly to help keep your postural alignment. Keep your back straight, body still, and your head level and looking straight ahead as you do the exercise.

Step 4: Relax the musculature of your chest and back. Close your eyes and once again visualize yourself actually doing the movement while focusing on the shoulder and trapezius muscles.

Step 5: Hold the dumbbells across your thighs and keep your palms facing toward your body. Focus on the muscles of the shoulder including the trapezius muscles which run across your upper back. Although you will be pulling the weight up with your hands, you must let the elbows lead the motion, keeping them high as you pull up.

Step 6: Begin pulling the weight up slowly, concentrating on feeling the stimulation of the focused muscles. Lead with your elbows, and lift the dumbbells to a point where they come close to the height of your chin. The most important thing to do at this position of the exercise is to consciously focus on and physically contract the muscles of the trapezius.

Step 7: Slowly lower the dumbbells while maintaining the same exact form and posture you did when pulling up. When you reach the bottom (start) position, slowly begin pulling the weights back to the top position of the exercise using a controlled, fluid motion. Make sure that you do not jerk or use momentum to lift the dumbbells at any time during this exercise.

Dumbbell Upright Row

SECONDARY TARGET MUSCLES: **Biceps**

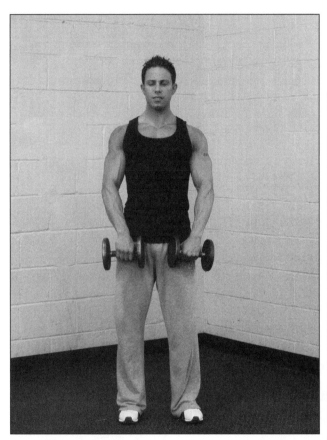

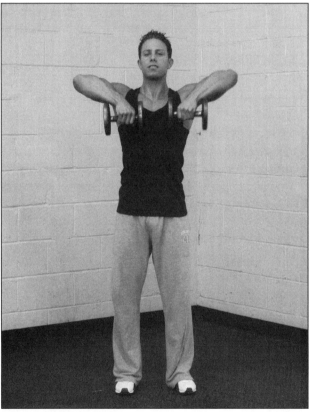

Mind Over Muscle Re-**MIND**-er:

Use your breath to do more than just deliver oxygen to your muscles. When resting between sets, inhale through your nose and take in positive energy from the universe. When you go back to work, expend that positive energy with a forceful exhalation. You'll be surprised how much harder your muscles work when you connect them with that mental breath energy. Make sure not to hold the bar too close to your body, as this can injure the rotator cuff muscles. Hold the bar about 6 inches away from your body as you pull the bar upward.

Dumbbell Shrug

PRIMARY TARGET MUSCLES: Trapezius

NOTES: The trapezius can handle surprisingly heavy weights, so shoulder presses and other deltoid exercises don't even come close to the weights necessary for stimulating these powerful muscles across the top of your back. Nonetheless, begin with relatively light weights to get used to the form and work your way up. Dumbbells allow for a neutral grip instead of an overhand grip.

EXECUTION AND FORM

Step 1: Deadlift the weight to a standing position with your arms hanging straight down. Your feet should be shoulder width apart and your knees pointing forward with a slight bend. Hold the dumbbells in a neutral grip and keep your arms straight at your sides.

Step 2: Throughout the exercise keep your back erect and your head straight and looking forward or with the chin tucked slightly. Your shoulders should be back, relaxed, and in line with your ears.

Step 3: Isometrically contract your traps, which connect your shoulders to the spine.

Step 4: Concentrating on the contraction, shrug your shoulders as if you were going to touch them to your ears. Don't let your head come forward as this will recruit the lats instead of isolating the traps.

Step 5: At the top of the shrug, squeeze your trapezius muscles hard. Then slowly lower the weight to where your traps feel a comfortable stretch.

Step 6: Without stopping or using momentum, contract the traps and start the shoulders back up to the top in a fluid motion.

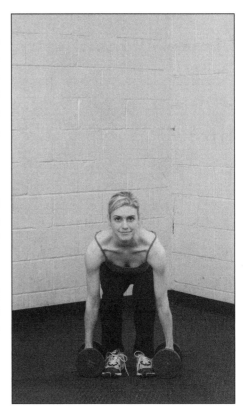

Dumbbell Shrug

SECONDARY TARGET MUSCLES: **Back**

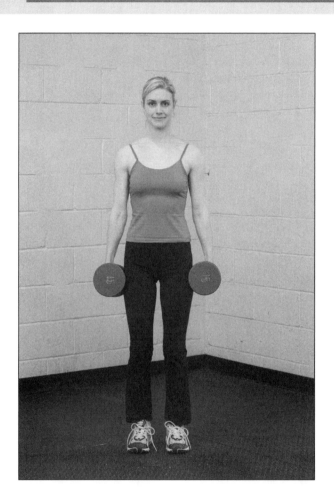 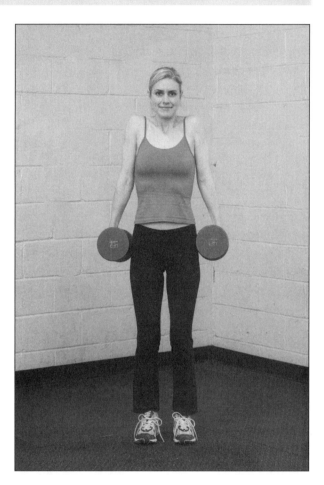

Mind Over Muscle Re-**MIND**-er:

Before picking up the dumbbells at the start of a set, assume your working stance and tense up your entire body from head to toe as if you were going to use the Full Body Tension technique. Doing so prepares your body for action and bearing the weight. Maintain the tension as you pick up the dumbbells and tense with them for a moment before beginning the set. Just before starting the first rep, switch your attention and tensing to the trapezius, allowing other muscles to relax. Imagine shrugging your shoulders so high, that you can touch your ears. This will ensure optimum muscle fiber recruitment in the trapezius muscles.

Smith Machine Shrug

PRIMARY TARGET MUSCLES: Trapezius

NOTES: The trapezius can handle surprisingly heavy weights, so shoulder presses and other deltoid exercises don't even come close to the weights necessary for stimulating these powerful muscles across the top of your back. Shrugs allow you to isolate the trapezius and hit them heavy. Nonetheless, begin with relatively light weights to get used to the form and work your way up. The Smith Machine allows you to use really heavy weights without spending the energy to lift them off the floor.

EXECUTION AND FORM

Step 1: Rack the bar at a height just below your hands when you are standing erect. Load the bar, starting with a weight that allows you to practice perfect form. Stand in front of the bar and lift it into an erect position with an overhand grip.

Step 2: Throughout the exercise, keep your back erect and your head straight and looking forward or with the chin tucked slightly. Your shoulders should be back, relaxed, and in line with your ears.

Step 3: Isometrically contract your traps, which connect your shoulders to the spine.

Step 4: Concentrating on the contraction, shrug your shoulders as if you were going to touch them to your ears. Don't let your head come forward, as this will recruit the lats instead of isolating the traps.

Step 5: At the top of the shrug, squeeze your trapezius muscles hard. Then slowly lower the weight to where your traps feel a comfortable stretch.

Step 6: Without stopping or using momentum, contract the traps and start the shoulders back up to the top in a fluid motion.

Smith Machine Shrug

SECONDARY TARGET MUSCLES: **Back**

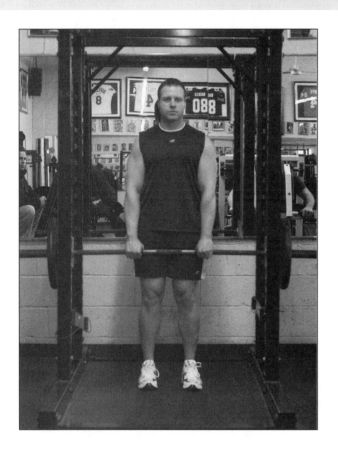
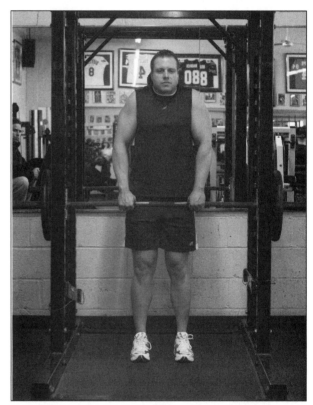

Mind Over Muscle Re-**MIND**-er:

To help establish the mind-to-muscle connection before every set, stand ready to pick up the weight but pause before doing so. During the pause, visualize yourself someplace peaceful: at a lake, on a mountain top, someplace quiet and familiar. Let the peacefulness of that vision sink into your head and your muscles. Relax and empty your thoughts for the day. Then methodically tense each muscle in your body in turn, ending with the traps or whatever muscle you're about to exercise.

Barbell Shoulder Press

PRIMARY TARGET MUSCLES: Deltoids (medial, anterior, posterior)

NOTES: Unlike behind-the-neck presses, which risk damaging the rotator cuffs, shoulder presses are a great exercise to develop all three heads of the shoulder or deltoid muscles. A narrower grip focuses more on the muscles of the medial and rear deltoids with an emphasis on the triceps. A wider grip incorporates the front and medial deltoids. Use a weight light enough to allow a full range of motion; you should bring the bar down very close to your upper chest muscles.

EXECUTION AND FORM

Step 1: Take a seat with your back fully upright and place your feet flat on the floor in front of you. Your knees should also be facing straight ahead and the racked barbell should be at forehead level and SLIGHTLY in front of you. If your seat is too far from the bar, you risk injuring your lower back or overstressing your shoulders and arms while unracking the bar. If you're not using a rack, have someone hand you the barbell after you sit down.

Step 2: Take hold of the barbell with your grip of choice. Remember that grip variation will stimulate different muscles; assess your shoulder muscles and choose a grip that targets the deltoid heads that need further development.

Step 3: As you hold the bar, make sure that your arms and elbows are as wide as possible—as if you were trying to touch your elbows behind your back. Keep your forearms perpendicular to the floor and your head and neck relaxed at all times through the movement. Never turn your head while doing any of these exercises—you could seriously injure yourself.

Step 4: Before lifting, close your eyes and visualize yourself doing the movement. Focus on the shoulder muscles you are about to stimulate. Pay particular attention to the deltoid head (medial, anterior, or posterior) that needs the most development.

Step 5: Pick up the bar and begin the exercise from the top position. Get a spotter's help in unracking the bar if you need to.

Step 6: From the overhead position, squeeze the bar tightly with your hands and slowly lower the bar to just under the chin. The upper arm, from the elbow to the shoulder, should end up slightly below parallel to the floor, with your forearms perpendicular to the ceiling.

Step 7: Slowly begin pressing upward in a controlled, fluid motion, without resting. Make sure that you do not use any momentum. Stay focused on the movement of your shoulder muscles. A common mistake is to stick the chest way out when pressing up. Doing this takes primary stimulation away from the shoulder muscles and directs it to the chest muscles. Relax the chest at all times during this exercise. If you see your chest rise or feel your chest muscles handling the majority of the work, stop and correct yourself. You may either be going too heavy, or you just need to practice your form without weight.

Step 8: When you reach the top of the movement, do not lock out the

Barbell Shoulder Press

SECONDARY TARGET MUSCLES: **Triceps**

elbow joint. Doing so shifts all of the weight from the shoulders to the elbow joint, thus interrupting muscle stimulation. This can hurt the elbow joint and limit shoulder muscle stimulation.

Step 9: From this point, hold the extended position, then slowly lower the bar in a smooth, controlled, fluid motion, without resting.

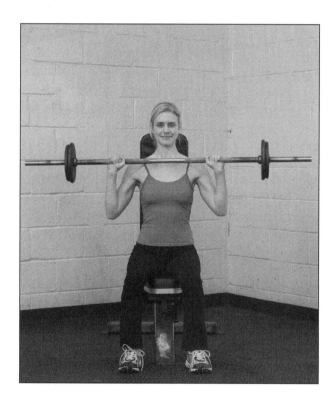
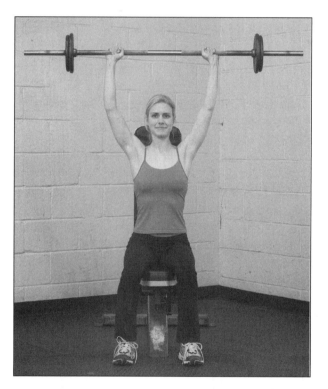

Mind Over Muscle Re-MIND-er:

Roger Bannister, the first person to run a mile in less than four minutes, did his running workouts with a slip of paper in his shoe that read "3:58." That's not a Bible verse; that was his goal: 3 minutes, 58 seconds. With every step he was reminded of his goal. Try it for yourself; write your fitness goal on a piece of paper and put it where you can see it during your set.

Dumbbell Shoulder Press

PRIMARY TARGET MUSCLES: Deltoids (medial, anterior, posterior)

NOTES: Unlike behind-the-neck presses, which risk damaging the rotator cuffs, shoulder presses are a great exercise to develop all three heads of the shoulder or deltoid muscles. Use a weight light enough to allow a full range of motion; you should bring the dumbbells down to a level where the backs of the arms are parallel to the floor.

EXECUTION AND FORM

Step 1: Take a seat with your back fully upright and place your feet flat on the floor in front of you. Your knees should also be facing straight ahead.

Step 2: Either lift your dumbbells to the shoulders before sitting, or put them on your thighs and use your knees to lift them to the shoulder like the Incline Bench Press. Keep your forearms perpendicular to the floor—if you let the dumbbells get too far apart, the weight can quickly get out of control because there is no bar holding them together and the risk of injury is huge.

Step 3: As you hold the dumbbells, make sure that your arms and elbows are as wide as possible—as if you were trying to touch your elbows behind your back. Keep your head and neck relaxed at all times through the movement. Never turn your head while doing any of these exercises—you could end up seriously injured.

Step 4: Before lifting, close your eyes and visualize yourself doing the movement. Focus on the shoulder muscles you are about to stimulate. Pay particular attention to the deltoid head (medial, anterior, or posterior) that needs the most development.

Step 5: From the overhead position, squeeze the dumbbell handles tightly with your hands and slowly lower them to chest level. The upper arm, from the elbow to the shoulder, should end up slightly below parallel to the floor, with your forearms perpendicular to the ceiling.

Step 6: Slowly begin pressing upward in a controlled, fluid motion, without resting. Make sure that you do not use any momentum. Stay focused on the movement of your shoulder muscles. A common mistake is to stick the chest way out when pressing up. Doing this takes primary stimulation away from the shoulder muscles and directs it to the chest muscles. Relax the chest at all times during this exercise. If you see your chest rise or feel your chest muscles handling the majority of the work, stop and correct yourself. You may either be going too heavy, or you just need to practice your form with less weight.

Step 7: When you reach the top of the movement, do not lock out the elbow joint. Doing so shifts all of the weight from the shoulders to the elbow joint, thus interrupting muscle stimulation. This can hurt the elbow joint and limit shoulder muscle stimulation.

Step 8: From this point, hold the extended position and then slowly lower the dumbbells in a controlled, fluid motion, without resting.

Dumbbell Shoulder Press

SECONDARY TARGET MUSCLES: **Triceps**

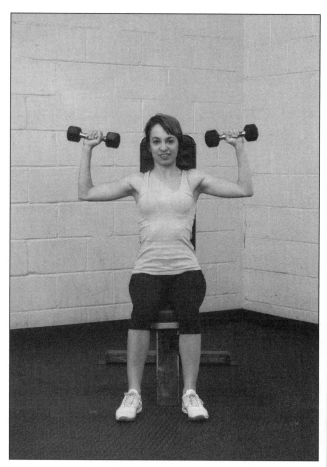
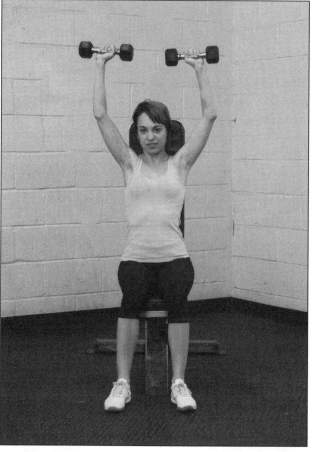

Mind Over Muscle Re-MIND-er:

Use the Full Body Tension Technique. This prepares the body for action. Maintain the tension as you pick up the dumbbells and tense with them for a moment before beginning the set. Just before starting the first rep, switch your attention and tensing to the shoulders.

Handstand Press

PRIMARY TARGET MUSCLES: Deltoids (medial, anterior, posterior)

NOTES: The handstand press is a good replacement for shoulder presses when you are traveling or don't have access to gym weights. However, if you find that you are unable to press your own body weight, I recommend you do shoulder presses with a substitute weight, such as a heavy suitcase or duffel bag.

EXECUTION AND FORM

Step 1: Do a handstand with your back and heels against a wall, making sure to do this in a location in which nothing will get damaged—including yourself—if you lose your balance.

Step 2: Lower your body toward the floor, but stop just short of touching the floor with your head.

Step 3: Raise your body as if you are doing a shoulder press with the floor. Make sure that you do not use any momentum. Stay focused on the movement of your shoulder muscles. A common mistake is to stick the chest way out when pressing up. Doing this takes primary stimulation away from the shoulder muscles and directs it to the chest muscles. Relax the chest at all times during this exercise. If you see your chest rise or feel your chest muscles handling the majority of the work, stop and correct yourself.

Handstand Press

SECONDARY TARGET MUSCLES: **Triceps**

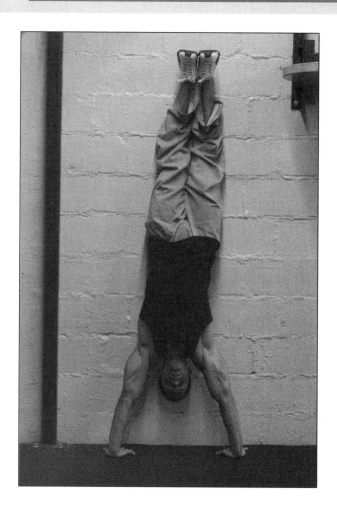

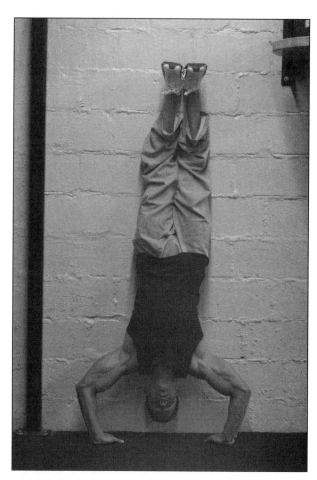

Mind Over Muscle Re-MIND-er:

Handstands are a great exercise even if you can't handstand press your body weight. Just practicing a handstand against a wall will help you improve balance. As you become accustomed to doing handstands, bend your elbows and do either partial reps or hold a partial-rep position. This will strengthen your shoulders and gradually move you toward the ability to do a full handstand press. Like all exercises, this creates something called neural tracing on the brain, which will help establish new and long-lasting brain (mind/muscle) connections.

Dumbbell Lateral Raise

PRIMARY TARGET MUSCLES: Deltoid Medial Head

NOTES: Leave your ego outside the gym and use a low weight that allows you to concentrate on perfect form—it's very easy to get too much weight on this exercise because the dumbbells are held so far from your body. If you pick a weight that is too heavy, momentum will force muscles other than the shoulder to do the work. Some people have the tendency to bend at the elbows, but keeping them straight isolates the medial deltoid better.

EXECUTION AND FORM

Step 1: Take a standing position with a shoulder width stance. Align the body from the bottom up, beginning with the feet. Make sure the feet are pointing straight ahead. Keep the knees pointing straight ahead and slightly bent to help avoid any unnecessary back strain.

Step 2: Hold a dumbbell in each hand with arms straight down at your sides. Your palms should be pointed toward your body in a neutral grip.

Step 3: Focus your attention on the medial deltoid muscle and contract it.

Step 4: Keeping your arms straight and at the sides of your body, lift the weights directly out to the sides until they reach the level of your cheeks.

Step 5: As you lift the dumbbells, your palms should face downward, so your shoulder muscles rather than the biceps muscles do the work.

Step 6: At the top, squeeze your delts and hold the weights there for a moment.

Step 7: While maintaining your posture and body alignment, lower the dumbbells in a controlled fashion back to the starting point.

Dumbbell Lateral Raise

SECONDARY TARGET MUSCLES: Deltoid Anterior, Deltoid Posterior

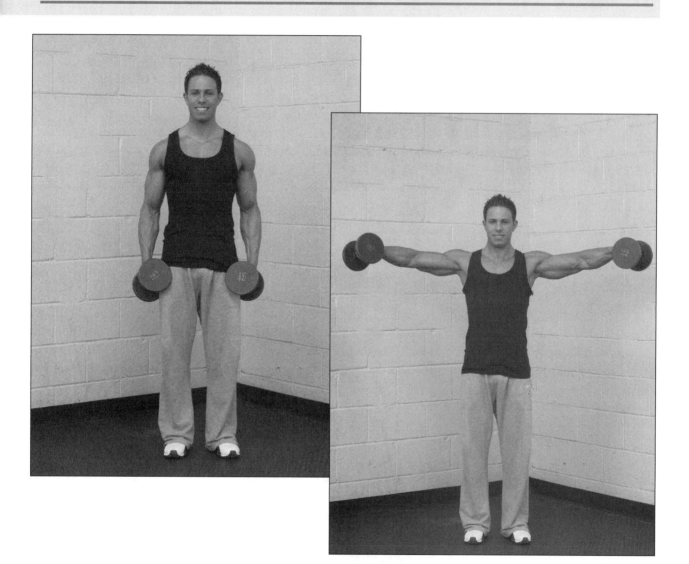

Mind Over Muscle Re-**MIND**-er:

Before each exercise, take time to visualize yourself performing the exercise perfectly. It should be a detailed vision that includes how it looks, how you're standing, how it feels, and every other aspect you can envision. This visualization prepares the mind and body to duplicate what you've imagined. It's like programming your system for success.

Bent-Over Lateral Raise

PRIMARY TARGET MUSCLES: Posterior Deltoid

NOTES: The rear or posterior deltoid is one of the most neglected muscles in the body. By using this exercise to develop this muscle, you will give your shoulders a fantastic three-dimensional look. There are three ways to execute this exercise:

1. Seated on a flat bench with your chest bent over your knees
2. Seated backward on an incline bench with your chest against the back rest
3. Standing while bent at the hips and your back parallel to the floor. When using this method, be sure to keep your knees slightly bent so you don't put too much strain on your back.

Be careful not to involve your lower back. Doing so may lead to injury. Instead of thinking that you are lifting the dumbbells, think that you are squeezing your shoulder blades together and spreading the dumbbells apart. This will keep your focus on the rear deltoids where it should be.

EXECUTION AND FORM

Step 1:
- **FLAT BENCH VERSION:** Hold a dumbbell in each hand and let your arms hang at your sides as you take a seat facing backward on the incline bench, with your legs straddling the backrest. Rest your entire torso, from your pelvic bone to your chest, on the incline bench's angled pad with your head and eyes looking straight ahead.
- **FLAT BENCH VERSION (pictured):** Your legs should straddle the bench with your knees facing forward and your shins perpendicular to the floor. Bend at the hips and nearly touch your chest to your knees.
- **STANDING VERSION:** Bend your knees and bend over at the hips

until your back is parallel to the floor or a little higher.

Step 2: Position your feet shoulder width apart, pointing them straight ahead at all times during the exercise. Make sure that your knees are bent so there is no unnecessary lower back stress.

Step 3: With your palms facing each other, keep looking straight ahead. As you prepare to do the exercise, focus all of your attention and concentration on the rear deltoid muscles of the shoulder. Know where these muscles are located and how they feel when stimulated. This is why we suggest that you go light, so that you may isolate these muscles without incorporating others into the movement.

Step 4: Slowly and without momentum, begin lifting the dumbbells out to each side of your body. As you lift the dumbbells to the sides of your body, your elbows will be leading the motion, but keep them locked at a nearly straight angle. If you lead the movement with the dumbbells you'll take all of the focus off the rear deltoid muscles.

Step 5: Do not lift your torso as you lift. If you find that you are in fact lifting with your back for momentum, stop! Either lighten the weight or rest for a minute and do your next set. Don't just go through the motions only concerned with getting the weights up. Focus on isolation of the rear deltoid muscles, and make them contract hard.

Bent-Over Lateral Raise

SECONDARY TARGET MUSCLES: Trapezius

Step 6: Make sure that you lift the dumbbells straight out to your sides rather than behind you or out in front of you. Bringing the dumbbells behind shifts the focus to the trapezius muscles, and holding them forward shifts it to the front deltoids.

Step 7: Maintain your postural alignment and bring the dumbbells up to level with your shoulders or slightly higher. Squeeze the dumbbells up while you contract the rear deltoid muscles as hard as you can. Hold this contraction for a moment.

Step 8: Slowly begin lowering the dumbbells, making sure that you make the rear deltoid muscles continue to work during the lowering portion of the exercise.

Step 9: As you reach the bottom position, do not rest. Once again, slowly lift the dumbbells out to each side of your body in a smooth, controlled and fluid motion, without using momentum.

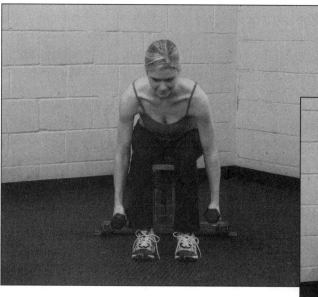
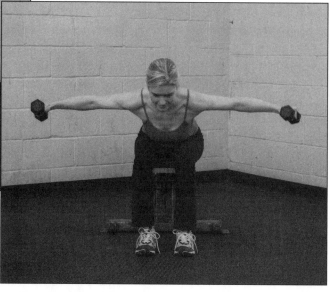

Mind Over Muscle Re-MIND-er:

Imagine that there is a string attached to each of the dumbbells. When the going gets tough, imagine someone above you pulling the strings to support you.

Rear Deltoid Machine

PRIMARY TARGET MUSCLES: Posterior Deltoid

NOTES: The seated rear delt machine gives you the ability to really focus on isolating the rear delts without the possibility of lower back injury and the burden of having to bend over at the hips. This is a perfect exercise for those who feel dizzy when bent over or feel too much chest compression from having to lean on the incline bench, or have lower back problems.

EXECUTION AND FORM

Step 1: Seat yourself on the machine and position your body so that you are sitting upright with your chest flush against the vertical pad. There should be a seat adjustment that will allow you to raise and lower the seat. Bring the seat to a height where your chin can rest neutrally on the edge of the pad in front of you. This is a good height to optimize the proper anatomical position for this shoulder exercise.

Step 2: Keep your feet flat on the floor and pointing straight ahead during the movement. Also, keep your knees pointing straight ahead at all times. On most rear delt machines, you will find inner thigh pads for added stability. Keep your thighs snug against the pads to give you the added support needed to secure your core musculature.

Step 3: This machine is often used as a pec deck and gives you the option of adjusting the arm bars to your liking. For this particular exercise, you

will want the arm bars brought to the back position so they are just about touching one another. You also might have the option of taking your hand-grip in a palms facing position or an over-hand position. Take the over-hand position since this will take much stress off the wrists and allow better muscle control and isolation of the rear shoulders.

Step 4: Make sure that you keep a slight bend in the elbows at all times. This bend of the arms will help make sure that you keep the focus of resistance on the rear delts and off the triceps. You might reach a level of fatigue where you are forced to use the triceps muscles to move the weight. When you reach this point, either resist the temptation or simply lower the weight.

Step 5: Keep your sternum against the chest pad at all times during the exercise with your torso totally upright.

Step 6: Before you begin the movement, make sure you are consciously focused on the rear deltoid muscles and begin to isometrically contract them before moving the weight. This might take some practice to perfect, but you will soon multiply your muscle isolation abilities ten-fold.

Step 7: Begin pulling the bars away from each other while focusing on contracting your rear delts. Maintain your body alignment at all times. Imagine opening a pair of heavy doors. Bring the bars as far back as possible without jerking or using momentum to do so.

Step 8: When you reach the top of the movement, with arms fully extended outwards, hold this position and feel the rear shoulder muscles taking the brunt of the resistance. At this point, really squeeze the rear delts.

Step 9: Slowly allow the arms to return to the start position, resisting the bars on the negative portion of

Rear Deltoid Machine

SECONDARY TARGET MUSCLES: None

the exercise by continuing to keep the delts tense and contracted.

Step 10: Once you have reached the position where the bars are just about touching each other, do not allow the weight stack to touch the bottom. You want to keep constant tension on the muscles and must stop right before the weights touch bottom. From here immediately begin to bring the bars apart once again with great form.

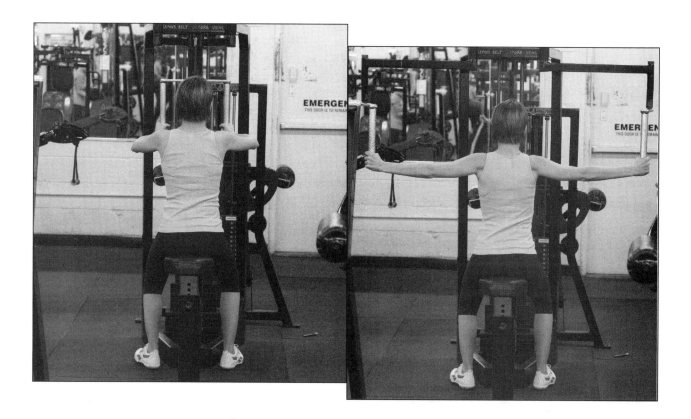

Mind Over Muscle Re-MIND-er:

When the going gets tough, turn on the nitro! Some street racers equip their cars with a tank of nitrous oxide—a high-octane fuel that gives the engine a sudden and powerful burst of speed that launches the car down the road. Energize your last reps in the set by mentally turning on your human nitro, adrenaline, and you'll get a burst of power to finish the set.

Isometric Lateral Raise

PRIMARY TARGET MUSCLES: Deltoid Medial Head

NOTES: Isometric Lateral Raises can be done one arm at a time with isometric exercises. They are a good replacement for Dumbbell Lateral Raises when you don't have access to dumbbells.

EXECUTION AND FORM

Step 1: Stand next to a wall or other stationary object. The arm you're about to work should face the wall or object.

Step 2: With feet together, begin to do a lateral raise as if you were holding a dumbbell, but use the wall or object to isometrically resist the movement. Hold the contraction for the duration of the rep.

Step 3: Once you've completed a set with one arm, turn around and do the same with the other arm. Alternatively, use your non-working arm to resist the working arm by grabbing the forearm and pulling it toward the body.

Isometric Lateral Raise

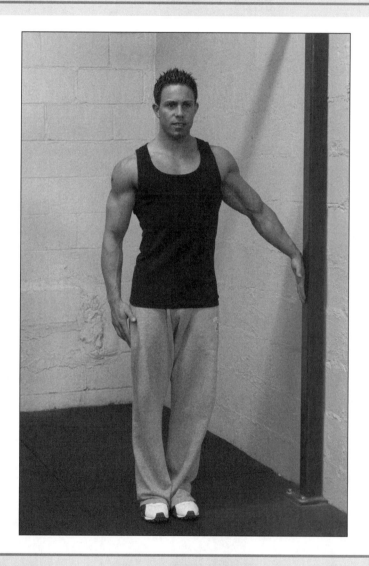

Mind Over Muscle Re-MIND-er:

Brain health and physical fitness go hand in hand. Being alert with good motor-memory skills will improve your workouts and help you build muscle more effectively. But the act of exercising, particularly when concentrating on the exercise, also stimulates and improves memory and other mental functions. It's a snowball effect that results in both enormous physical and mental well being.

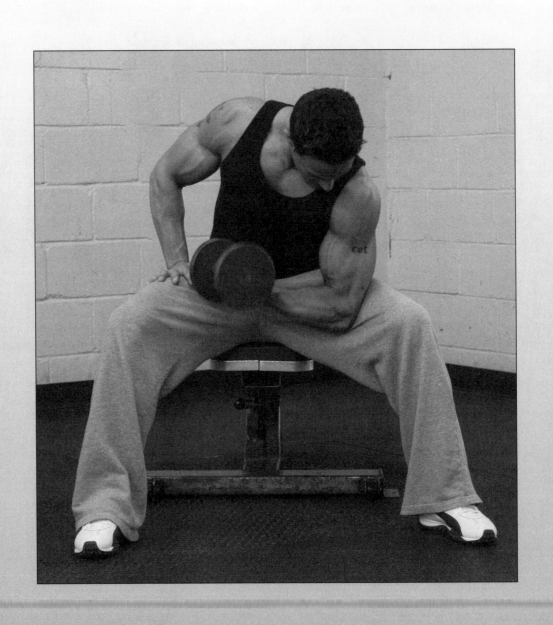

Arms

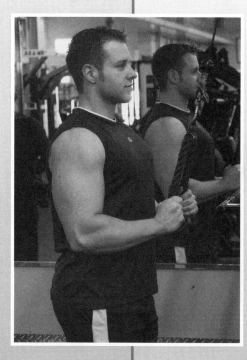

- Barbell Curl

- Wide Grip Barbell Curl

- Reverse E-Z Curl

- Hammer Curl

- Preacher Curl

- Dumbbell Concentration Curl

- Incline Dumbbell Curl

- High Pulley Biceps Curl

- Close Grip Bench Press

- Lying Dumbbell Triceps Extension

- Overhead Dumbbell Extension

- Overhead Rope Triceps Extension

- Dumbbell Triceps Kickback

- Pulley Triceps Kickback

- Triceps Pushdown

- Machine Triceps Extension

- Isometric Bicep Curl and Triceps Extension

MIND OVER MUSCLE

Barbell Curl

PRIMARY TARGET MUSCLES: **Biceps**

NOTES: This is the most basic of the biceps exercises and does an excellent job of developing the overall size of the biceps. Barbell curls can be done with either a straight bar or an E-Z Curl or cambered bar. The E-Z Curl bar allows you to lift heavier weight with less stress on the wrists than straight bar curls. If you have a pending strain such as tennis elbow or tendonitis, I recommend E-Z Curl bar curls over straight bar curls.

EXECUTION AND FORM

Step 1: Stand with your feet shoulder width apart and point them straight ahead. Using a palms-up grip with your hands approximately shoulder width apart, hold the bar across your thighs. Next, bend your knees slightly.

Step 2: Slightly contract the abdominal muscles. Stand straight up and stay that way throughout the movement. Stick your chest out and keep the shoulders back, which will help you maintain a straight back.

Step 3: Keep your head level and do not move it from that position for the rest of the exercise.

Step 4: Lock your elbows to the sides of your body and focus your attention on the biceps. Flex them a few times before lifting. Then squeeze the biceps and curl the bar up toward your shoulders in an arc-like motion.

Step 5: Keep the elbows pointing directly to the ground as you curl upward to avoid involving the shoulder muscles. As you curl upward, concentrate and focus all of your attention on the biceps muscles and feel them contract.

Step 6: As you reach the top of the movement, with the bar close to

your shoulders, contract the biceps muscles as hard as you possibly can.

Step 7: Slowly lower the bar while making sure that the biceps resist the weight on the way down. Stay focused on the biceps.

Step 8: As you reach the start position with the arms fully straightened, do not rest. Begin curling the bar once again in a smooth, controlled, and fluid motion without using momentum.

Barbell Curl

SECONDARY TARGET MUSCLES: **Inner Forearm**

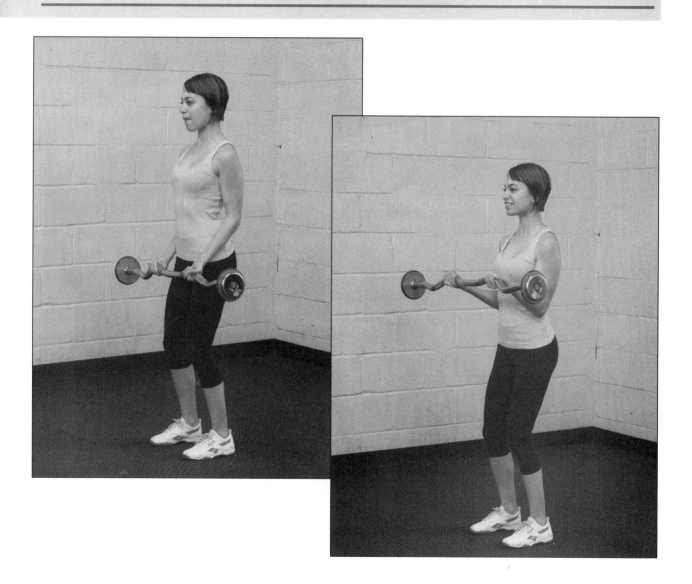

Mind Over Muscle Re-**MIND**-er:

When your curl reps get tough, contract your triceps isometrically before and during a repetition to give your biceps permission to unleash all their power!

Wide Grip Barbell Curl

PRIMARY TARGET MUSCLES: Biceps

NOTES: The wide grip barbell curl develops the inner biceps more, whereas the shoulder width grip works the outer bicep more. Wide grip curls are best done with a straight barbell rather than the E-Z bar.

EXECUTION AND FORM

Step 1: Stand with your feet shoulder width apart and point them straight ahead. Using a palms-up grip with your hands approximately 2 to 4 inches wider than your shoulder width grip, hold the bar across your thighs. Next, bend your knees slightly.

Step 2: Slightly contract the abdominal muscles. Stand straight up and stay that way throughout the movement. Stick your chest out and keep the shoulders back, which will help you maintain a straight back.

Step 3: Keep your head level and do not move it from that position for the rest of the exercise.

Step 4: Lock your elbows to the sides of your body and focus your attention on the biceps. Flex them a few times before lifting. Then squeeze the biceps and curl the bar up toward your shoulders in an arc-like motion.

Step 5: Keep the elbows pointing directly to the ground as you curl upward to avoid involving the shoulder muscles. As you curl upward, concentrate and focus all of your attention on the biceps. Feel the muscles contracting as you curl the bar upward.

Step 6: As you reach the top of the movement with the bar close to your shoulders, contract the biceps muscles as hard as you possibly can.

Step 7: Slowly lower the bar while making sure that the biceps endure the negative resistance on the way down to the bottom position. Stay focused on the biceps.

Step 8: As you reach the start position with the arms fully straightened, do not rest. Begin curling the bar once again in a smooth, controlled, and fluid motion without using momentum.

Wide Grip Barbell Curl

SECONDARY TARGET MUSCLES: Inner Forearm

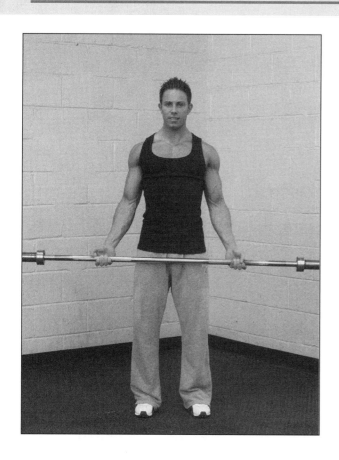

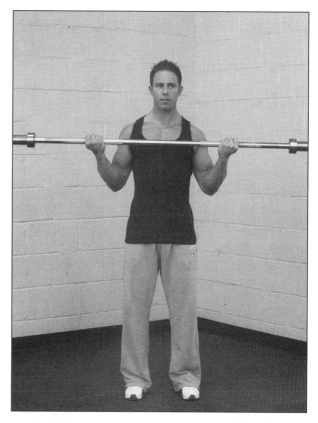

Mind Over Muscle Re-MIND-er:

When working your biceps think about scrunching the muscle up into a ball and squeezing it at the top of the curl. Visualize the muscle pulling together to make a softball size lump on your arm. This will take your mind off the difficulty of the set, train the muscle to contract tightly, and cause it to grow in an aesthetically appealing way. You might also want to try the Flushing technique here.

Reverse E-Z Curl

PRIMARY TARGET MUSCLES: **Brachialis (outer bicep)**

NOTES: The exercise alignment and execution is the same as that of curls using an E-Z bar, except that the hands are holding the bar with the palms facing the thighs on the outer handles of the bar for direct forearm stimulation.

EXECUTION AND FORM

Step 1: First, take your hand position by placing your hands with an overhand grip on the outer handles of the bar. Using a lighter weight than for standard barbell curls, hold the bar across your thighs with your palms facing your body. Stand with your feet shoulder width apart and point them straight ahead. Next, bend your knees slightly.

Step 2: Slightly contract the abdominal muscles. Stand straight up and stay that way throughout the movement. Stick your chest out and keep the shoulders back, which will help you maintain a straight back.

Step 3: Keep your head level and do not move it from that position for the rest of the exercise.

Step 4: Lock your elbows to the sides of your body and focus your attention on the outer biceps. Flex them a few times before lifting to develop the mind-muscle connection. Then squeeze the biceps and curl the bar up toward your shoulders in an arc-like motion.

Step 5: Keep the elbows pointing directly to the ground as you curl upward to avoid involving the shoulder muscles. As you curl upward, concentrate and focus all of your attention on the outer biceps muscles. Imagine those muscles are

steel cables reeling in two massive crane arms.

Step 6: As you reach the top of the movement with the bar close to your shoulders, contract the biceps muscles as hard as you possibly can.

Step 7: Slowly lower the bar while making sure that the biceps endure the negative resistance on the way down to the bottom position. Stay focused on the biceps.

Step 8: As you reach the start position with the arms fully straightened, do not rest. Begin curling the bar once again in a smooth, controlled, and fluid motion without using momentum.

Reverse E-Z Curl

SECONDARY TARGET MUSCLES: **Forearm**

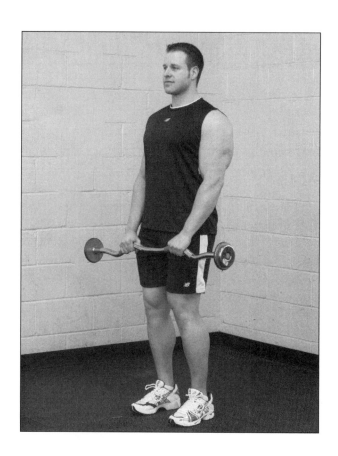
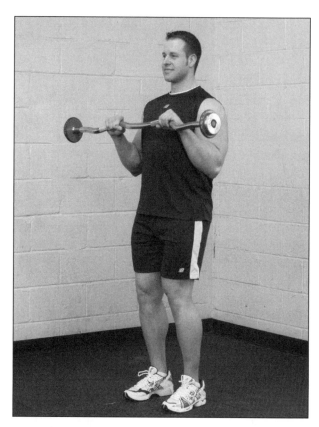

Mind Over Muscle Re-MIND-er:

Don't just think about your muscle during the concentric or lifting phase of a movement. Also get into that muscle during the eccentric or lowering phase. Feel each muscle fiber resist as you lower the weight. Experience the stretch of the muscle along the final length of the extension.

Hammer Curl

PRIMARY TARGET MUSCLES: Biceps (outer head)

NOTES: You can do this exercise either sitting, which will make it more strict, or standing, which will allow you to go a bit heavier. While I describe the standing version below, I suggest that you include both versions in your training routine.

EXECUTION AND FORM

Step 1: Choose two light dumbbells so that you can practice perfect form. With the dumbbells in hand, begin the alignment of your body by placing your feet about shoulder width apart and pointing straight ahead of you. Slightly bend the knees.

Step 2: Allow the dumbbells to hang down at your sides with your palms and dumbbells facing the sides of your body. Make sure that your elbows stay pointed at the ground at all times during the biceps curl exercise.

Step 3: Keep your upper body straight by contracting your abdominal muscles slightly, sticking out your chest and keeping your shoulder blades squared off. Keep your head level, and your eyes looking straight ahead. Standing against a wall will help you maintain your posture and isolate your biceps.

Step 4: Focus your attention on your biceps and give them a tight squeeze. Contract the biceps and curl the dumbbells up with palms and dumbbells facing each other. Your forearm and the dumbbell should look like a hammer about to drive a nail, which is where the exercise gets its name.

Step 5: Focus on driving the thumbs to your front shoulders, concentrating on feeling the biceps and forearm muscles working.

Step 6: Once you've reached the top position of the exercise, contract the biceps and forearm muscles as hard as you possibly can.

Step 7: From the top position, slowly and smoothly lower the dumbbells back to the starting position. As you reach the bottom of the exercise, the palms of your hands and dumbbells should remain facing each other and held to the sides of your body.

Step 8: Make sure that there is a smooth transition when switching directions from both the top position going into the lowering of the dumbbells, and also from the bottom position going into the curling or raising of the dumbbells. Both scenarios must be done with no rest in between either of the direction changes, unless you are so fatigued by the end of the set that you need a few seconds rest in order to get a couple more repetitions.

Hammer Curl

SECONDARY TARGET MUSCLES: **Forearm Extensors (brachio-radialis)**

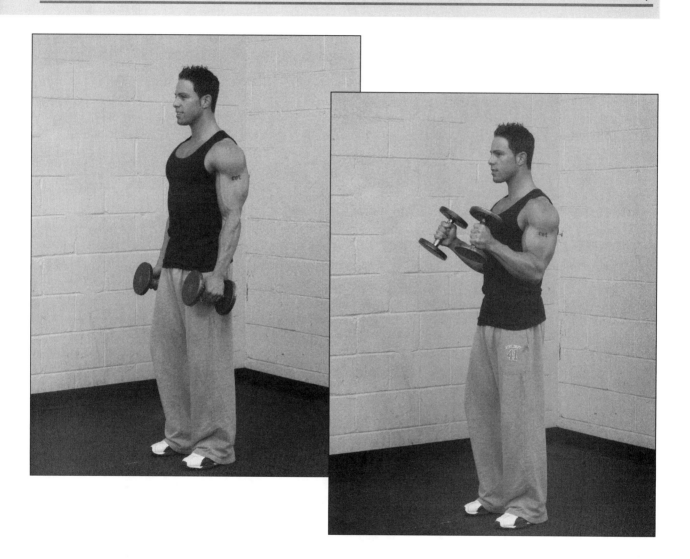

Mind Over Muscle Re-**MIND**-er:

Envision your arms and the dumbbells as those hammer-shaped pump arms on an oil well. Think about how they pump up and down all day long without a break in rhythm. Transfer the image to your arms as they pump that dumbbell up and down . . . up and down . . . up and down.

155

Preacher Curl

PRIMARY TARGET MUSCLES: Lower Biceps

NOTES: Preacher curls target the lower biceps, which don't get as much of a workout during standing barbell curls as do the upper biceps. By doing preacher curls you give the biceps a nice, rounded and complete appearance. They also take the strain off your lower back because you are seated at a bench. Preacher curls can be done with either a straight bar or an E-Z or cambered bar. The E-Z bar allows you to lift heavier weight with less stress on the wrists. If you have a pending strain such as tennis elbow or tendonitis, I recommend E-Z bar curls over straight bar curls. If your outer biceps need additional work, you can use a reverse or pronated grip with this exercise.

EXECUTION AND FORM

Step 1: Take a seat at the preacher bench, straddling the arm pad post with your legs. Put your chest against the close edge of the arm pad and rest your upper arms on top of the pad. Position yourself so the edge of the pad almost touches your armpits.

Step 2: Grip the barbell or E-Z bar with a supinated palms-up grip. Start with your triceps flat on the pad and your elbows slightly bent.

Step 3: Slightly contract the abdominal muscles. Keep your back straight and your head level throughout the exercise.

Step 4: Keep your head level and do not move it from that position for the rest of the exercise.

Step 5: Focus your attention on the biceps and flex them a few times before lifting. Then squeeze the biceps and curl the bar up toward your shoulders in an arc-like motion.

Step 6: Keep the elbows in place on the pad as you curl upward to avoid involving the shoulders muscles. As you curl upward, concentrate and focus all of your attention on the biceps muscles. Feel the muscles contracting as you curl the bar upward.

Step 7: Stop the curl when your forearms are just short of perpendicular. Isometrically contract the biceps.

Step 8: Slowly lower the bar while making sure the biceps resist the weight on the way down. Stay focused on the biceps.

Step 9: As you reach the start position, with the arms not quite fully straightened, do not rest. Begin curling the bar once again in a controlled and fluid motion without using momentum.

Preacher Curl

SECONDARY TARGET MUSCLES: Upper Biceps, Wrist

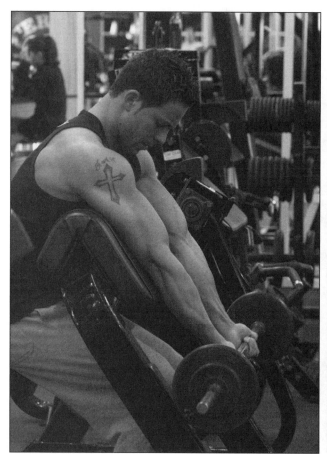

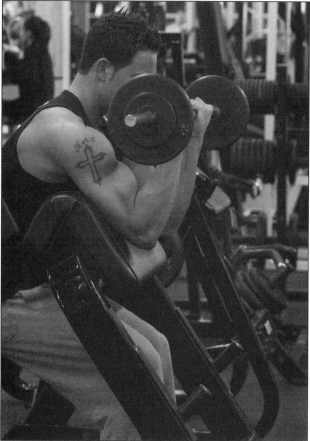

Mind Over Muscle Re-MIND-er:

Be your own coach. At least one study has shown that having someone coaching you on, with comments like "Come on!", "Keep it up!" and "Let's go!" will significantly increase the effort you give to the task at hand. Because these remarks are like commands, they trigger the instinct to do as commanded. Coming from yourself, you don't even have a good reason to buck authority. Try coaching yourself out loud with these and similar commands.

Dumbbell Concentration Curl

PRIMARY TARGET MUSCLES: **Biceps**

NOTES: This exercise is all about putting your mind into the muscle and focusing every bit of your attention on the exercise you are about to do. It will do wonders to heighten your biceps. Perform this exercise one arm at a time.

EXECUTION AND FORM

Step 1: You can do the concentration curl either in a sitting position or while standing. Whichever position you choose, bend over at the hips and take a dumbbell in one hand. As always, the dumbbell weight should be light at first so that you can practice perfect form.

Step 2: Sit at the edge of a bench and support your arm by resting your elbow on your thigh. If doing this from a standing position, bend your knees slightly and bend at the hips until your back is parallel to the floor. Let the arm with the dumbbell hang straight down while supporting your body weight with your opposite hand by placing it on your thigh.

Step 3: Do not curl the weight straight up to your chest. You must curl the weight with your arm angled in toward your body. This will help make certain that the exercise motion is correct, following the direction toward your shoulders rather than your chest. To start, bend over at the hips and fully extend the arm that you will be exercising while the other arm is resting on your thigh. Flex your bicep and feel how it works before beginning the lift.

Step 4: Squeeze the biceps and curl the weight toward your shoulder. At the top, contract the biceps muscle as hard as you possibly can, while keeping your arm pointing at the ground.

Step 5: Slowly lower the dumbbell back to the starting position, resisting the weight the entire way down. Feel the contraction as you lower the dumbbell.

Step 6: Without rest or momentum, once again squeeze the biceps and start curling the weight toward the shoulder with great focus and concentration. Once you have completed the desired amount of repetitions, switch arms and do the same amount of repetitions.

Dumbbell Concentration Curl

SECONDARY TARGET MUSCLES: **None**

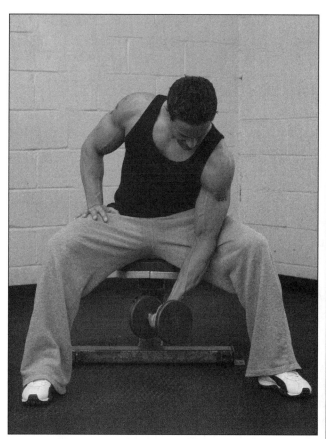

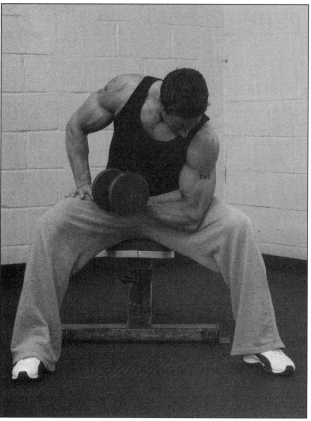

Mind Over Muscle Re-**MIND**-er:

With the dumbbell in hand, pause for a moment before beginning your first rep and concentrate on your breathing. Slow it down and breathe in the same rhythm you'll use to lift. Breathe in through your nose and out through your mouth. If you're using the "Two-Step Rep" scheme, exhale on a count of two, hold for two, and inhale for two. Start the curls by contracting on an exhale, hold on the hold, and lower on the inhale. By focusing on breathing you are able to concentrate more and give you muscles a rhythm to work to.

Incline Dumbbell Curl

PRIMARY TARGET MUSCLES: Biceps

NOTES: The incline dumbbell curl is a super exercise for developing great looking biceps. Due to the full stretch and range of motion of this exercise, it is designed to work the full length of the biceps with added emphasis on the outer head of the muscle. Because it requires strict form and isolation, you should start doing the exercise with a weight lighter than what you'd usually use for a regular dumbbell curl. Remember, form is everything. Make sure to avoid momentum and keep the form strict. Do not sacrifice good form for heavy weight (and ego)!

EXECUTION AND FORM

Step 1: Set an incline bench to a 45-degree angle.

Step 2: Pick two dumbbells with a weight that you can handle using perfect form. This exercise must be done very strictly in order to receive the desired effects.

Step 3: Sit down on the bench and rest the dumbbells on your thighs. Starting this way gives you some quality time to visualize and focus on the exercise you are about to do. This preparation can set up the proper mindset for even greater lifting performance.

Step 4: Lean all the way back into the bench so that your entire back is lying flat against the back pad. Stay that way for the entire exercise and do not take your back off the bench until the exercise is complete. Once you are properly positioned and ready to begin, take a firm grip on the dumbbells by squeezing the handles. Squeeze the biceps to lift the dumbbells off your thighs and lower them to hang at your sides.

Step 5: Make sure that your palms are facing the wall in front of you in a supinated grip for the entire exercise. Do not rotate your grip to a neutral grip on the descent as some weight lifters do.

Step 6: Keep your elbows pointed directly at the floor during the entire exercise. When people usually do any type of biceps curl, they allow their elbows to drift up with the curling movement, allowing the shoulders to flex forward. When this happens, the anterior shoulders become the prime movers of the weight being curled instead of the biceps, so be sure to avoid it.

Step 7: Once you are in position, focus all of your attention on the exercise you are about to do and on the biceps muscle itself. Begin curling the dumbbells at the same time, making sure that the elbows stay positioned toward the ground without moving upward as you curl.

Step 8: Curl the weights up until you can no longer curl while simultaneously contracting the biceps muscles as hard as you can.

Step 9: Slowly and smoothly lower the dumbbells until your arms are fully elongated and back at your sides.

Incline Dumbbell Curl

SECONDARY TARGET MUSCLES: **None**

Step 10: Without rest and without using any momentum, slowly and steadily begin curling the dumbbells back up toward your shoulders. If you jerk or in any way use momentum to begin curling the dumbbells, you risk serious injury to the biceps muscles.

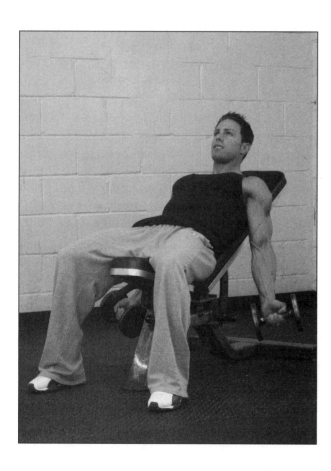

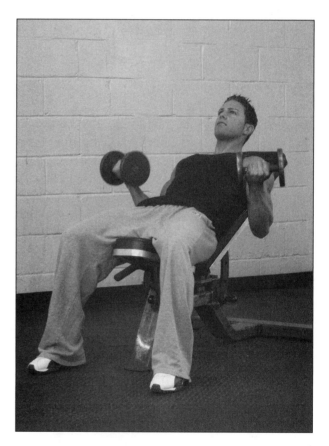

Mind Over Muscle Re-MIND-er:

Be aware of how far your muscles and joints are stretching at the bottom of an exercise. While a good stretch stimulates growth, stretching too far can cause stress and possibly damage muscles, tendons, and ligaments. Pay close attention to the signals from your body; it possesses an infinite wisdom, letting you know when you've gone too far.

High Pulley Biceps Curl

PRIMARY TARGET MUSCLES: Biceps

NOTES: Also known as the Crucifix Curl, the two-arm pulley biceps curl allows you to isolate the biceps from a unique angle and puts a sharp peak on top. It's essential to start with a light weight because your form can break down more quickly with heavier weights.

EXECUTION AND FORM

Step 1: Find a station where you can bring the cable attachment higher than you are or go to a lat pulldown station. Attach an EZ bar (cambered bar) to the hook and take either a close or wide underhand grip on the bar.

Step 2: Select a weight and position your body as follows: Feet should be hips width apart, knees slightly bent, abs tight, chest out shoulder back and relaxed downward.

Step 3: With arms fully extended, lean back and you'll feel a nice stretch in the biceps muscles.

Step 4: Contract your biceps isometrically and draw your concentration into the muscles. Tighten your abs and stabilize your body position as you begin to bring the bar towards your forehead. Throughout the movement, try to keep your elbows a bit tighter to your body. If the elbows float away, you will not be isolating your biceps.

Step 5: Do not allow the upper arm to move; all attempts to fully contract the biceps will depend on this.

Step 6: As you reach the point where the bar is close to your forehead, contract the biceps as hard as possible, hold and slowly come back to the starting, fully extended position. Without resting, bring your hands back toward your forehead for the desired number of repetitions.

High Pulley Biceps Curl

SECONDARY TARGET MUSCLES: Upper Chest

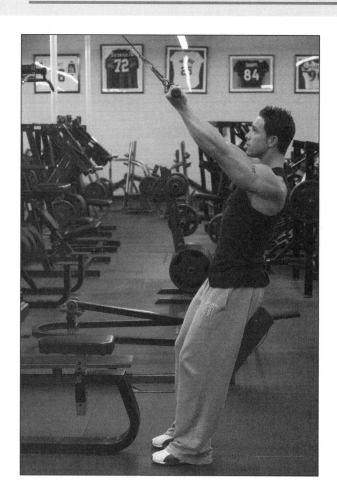

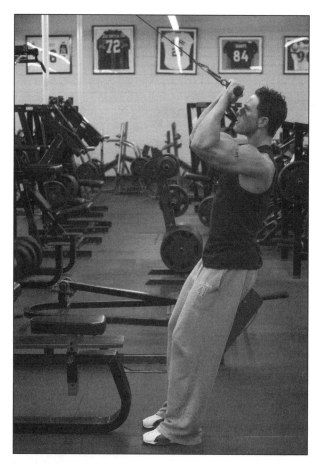

Mind Over Muscle Re-MIND-er:

Think about where you're feeling the contraction in this exercise. If you begin to feel your chest or shoulder muscles contracting, you're pulling your fists forward as well as inward. Try to touch the top of your shoulders and do not try to touch your fists together in front of you. Touching the fists in front of you will only recruit the muscles fibers of the chest.

Close Grip Bench Press

PRIMARY TARGET MUSCLES: **Triceps**

> **NOTES:** The conventional way to do the close grip bench press is with a barbell. It also calls for the arms to widen at the bottom, putting more emphasis on the inner chest muscles than the triceps. Our version of this exercise will be done with the E-Z curl bar and with a different arm position than the conventional version. This puts emphasis on the triceps with a secondary workload to the inner chest muscles.

EXECUTION AND FORM

Step 1: Sit on a flat bench and rest the loaded E-Z bar on the very top of your thighs and pull it tight to your hips and lower abdomen. Lie back on the bench, then slide or roll the bar up your body onto your chest. Alternately, you can have someone hand the bar to you when you are already lying down or rack it in a bench press rack until you are ready.

Step 2: Place your feet flat onto the floor and pointing straight ahead.

Step 3: Lift the bar into place by pressing it up using your chest muscles, just like the chest press. Hold it above your chest and keep it there. You will begin the exercise in this position to avoid stressing the elbow joint.

Step 4: Your arm, from shoulder to wrist, should form a straight line perpendicular to the floor. Your arms must stay close to your body and stay in a straight line. This is what will create primary isolation on the triceps muscles and allow better control of the bar.

Step 5: Take a position on the bar so that your hands are in the outer curved position of the bar. The inner curved position will create too much wrist strain. The proper spacing will be about 8 to 10 inches apart.

Step 6: Slowly lower the bar down as if you were lowering the bar during a bench press movement. Keep your arms riding closely to the sides of your body with your elbows bending toward your hips rather than bending outward. This technique is essential for proper triceps stimulation.

Step 7: Remember to consciously focus all of your attention on proper form and intense stimulation of the triceps during the movement.

Step 8: Continue to lower the bar in a controlled manner and bring the bar down to around mid-chest. Without resting, and without momentum, use your triceps muscles to push the bar off your chest and back to the start position. Remember to maintain your proper form with the arms riding close to the sides of your body.

Step 9: As you reach the top of the movement, squeeze the triceps muscles as hard as you can without locking out your elbow joints.

Step 10: Make sure that there is a smooth transition when switching directions from the top position going into the lowering of the bar, and also from the bottom position going into the extension or raising of the bar. There should be no rest at all when switching from the bottom position into the upward extension of the bar.

Close Grip Bench Press

SECONDARY TARGET MUSCLES: **Pectorals, Serratus**

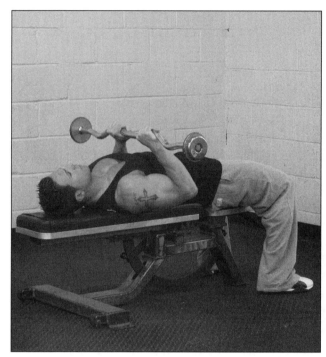

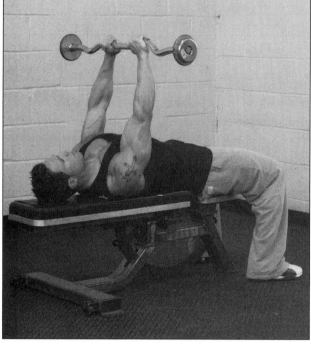

Mind Over Muscle Re-**MIND**-er:

When you're on your back pushing a weight to the sky, it's easy to think Bench Press and use your chest to push. Keep your mind on your triceps and focus on straightening your arms rather than pushing. Do your best to keep the elbows close to your body.

Lying Dumbbell Triceps Extension

PRIMARY TARGET MUSCLES: Triceps

NOTES: The lying position provides greater stability to lift more safely, preventing injury to your lower back. It also allows greater leverage to occur, much like the flat dumbbell press, allowing better strength output with a smoother exercise movement. Always make sure to move the dumbbells slowly from start to finish and squeeze the triceps muscles at the top of the movement to really feel those triceps working. It is a good idea to bring the elbows back, where the elbows point diagonally behind you versus straight up toward the ceiling. This slight slant backward will help to take some stress off of the elbow joint and transfer more of it to the triceps muscle.

EXECUTION AND FORM

Step 1: Pick up two dumbbells, making sure that they are light enough for you to practice perfect form. Sit at the end of a flat bench with the weights positioned upright on top of your thighs.

Step 2: It is very important to grip both dumbbell handles all the way at the end closest to your thighs. Make sure to slide your hands all the way to the bottom of the handle so that the pinky side of your hand is up against the weight plate. Doing this will help you control the weight better while also allowing you to contract the triceps harder at the top of the movement.

Step 3: Thrust each dumbbell up, just as you would when doing a dumbbell bench press, and lie back on the bench, placing your feet flat on the floor.

Step 4: As you are lying down, keeping the palms of your hands facing each other at all times, press the weights up using your chest muscles (chest press) to the fully-extended position. Begin the exercise in this position to avoid stressing the elbow joint. If you start at the bottom position of this exercise, you can easily create too much pressure on the elbow joint capsule and risk long-term injury. Remember, throughout the movement, your palms and inner elbows must always face each other. You want to make sure that your whole arm is in a direct line with your front shoulder (anterior deltoid). You must also make sure that your elbows are pointing diagonally behind you rather than directly at the ceiling during the exercise.

Step 5: Begin the exercise with the arms fully extended overhead, holding the dumbbells high to the ceiling. Once you are in the proper body alignment with the dumbbells overhead, contract your triceps intensely and slowly lower the dumbbells down toward your shoulders. Keep the elbows frozen in place at all times. These steps are necessary for proper triceps stimulation during this exercise. Remember to consciously focus all of your attention on proper form and stimulation of the triceps muscles.

Step 6: As you lower the dumbbells, stop just before the dumbbells reach your shoulders and begin to slowly and smoothly extend your arms from the elbows to the hands back

Lying Dumbbell Triceps Extension

SECONDARY TARGET MUSCLES: **Shoulders**

up to the starting position of the exercise. Remember to keep your upper arm frozen in place.

Step 7: As you reach the top of the exercise, contract the triceps muscles as hard as you possibly can for complete muscle stimulation. Make sure that you avoid excessively locking the elbow joint. Once you reach the position of full elbow extension, do not thrust the elbow joint into a locked position. Instead, contract the triceps muscles as hard as you possibly can. Practice using light weights with this technique as practice will make for perfect execution of the exercise and better results. Also, make sure that there is a smooth transition when switching directions from lowering the dumbbells to raising the dumbbells. Do not rest between lowering and raising the dumbbells.

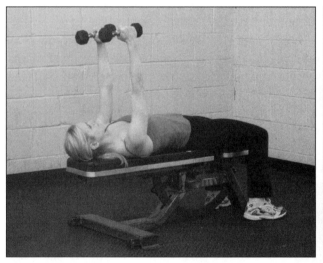
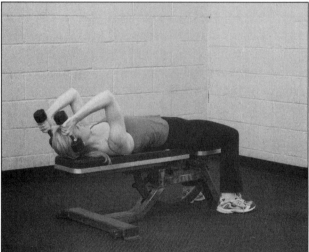

Mind Over Muscle Re-MIND-er:

It takes thorough rest and recuperation in order to be—and act—at your best. Lack of sleep will result in lack of concentration and scattered thinking—not to mention physical fatigue. These, of course, result in poor workouts and slower muscular gains. Be sure to get enough sleep and rest between workouts so you can keep your mind on what you're doing.

Overhead Dumbbell Extension

PRIMARY TARGET MUSCLES: Triceps (middle and inner heads)

NOTES: You can do this exercise either while seated or while standing. I recommend you do it seated as you will be less likely to cheat using momentum. Keep the elbows pointed to the ceiling above you at all times during the movement. This will help create a full range of motion for the triceps. You also need to hold the upper arms close to your head as you extend the weight overhead. Finally, pay attention to your handgrip on the dumbbell. If you fail to grip the dumbbell evenly, you may end up directing the force of the dumbbell resistance to one arm and ignore the other and create a muscle imbalance between the two arms. To fix this, you must learn to either grip the top, inner portion of the dumbbell with a separate, even grip for both hands or with an overlapping grip, having one hand overlap the other. Switch the overlapping hand between sets.

EXECUTION AND FORM

Step 1: Choose a weight that is light enough to practice perfect form, but heavy enough to benefit both arms. Place the dumbbell on top of your thigh. You can also have someone hand the dumbbell to you from behind. This is especially useful when using very heavy weight to avoid injuring the shoulder joints.

Step 2: Sit on a bench with a 90-degree angled back pad. Sit all the way back into the seat, making sure that your back is flat against the pad at all times during the movement.

Step 3: Before lifting the weight into position overhead, make sure that your feet are placed flat on the floor and pointed straight ahead. Make sure that your knees are also pointing straight ahead. Keep the head level and facing straight ahead at all times during the movement.

Step 4: Position the dumbbell overhead or have someone hand it to you from behind. Grasp the dumbbell with your grip of choice. If you find one hand has a dominant grip over the other, switch the hand in the dominant position between sets so your arms get a balanced workout.

Step 5: Point your elbows straight to the ceiling above you while holding your arms and elbows close to your head for triceps isolation.

Step 6: With the dumbbell overhead and in position, contract your triceps tightly and lower the dumbbell, while keeping the elbows pointed directly to the ceiling. It is important to do this because it isolates the triceps muscle and provides a full range of productive motion. It will also help you avoid hitting the dumbbell on the back of your head while extending and lowering the dumbbell.

Step 7: As you lower the dumbbell, focus on the triceps muscle and feel the stretch. Always take this negative portion slowly, remember to visualize, and stay in control. Pay close attention to the contraction of your triceps.

Step 8: Lower the dumbbell to a point where your forearms are slightly below parallel to the ground. You should feel a big stretch in the triceps.

Step 9: Without any rest and avoiding the use of momentum, squeeze the triceps and press the weight back up to the top position. Keep your elbows locked in place and your body in correct alignment.

Step 10: All of your attention must be on the triceps muscle, focusing on the isolation of the muscles. As you approach the top of the movement, contract the triceps muscles as hard as you possibly can while avoiding intensely locking out the elbow joints.

Overhead Dumbbell Extension

SECONDARY TARGET MUSCLES: **Triceps (outer head)**

Step 11: Hold this contraction for a two-second count and begin your descent, lowering the dumbbell in a slow, controlled, and fluid manner.

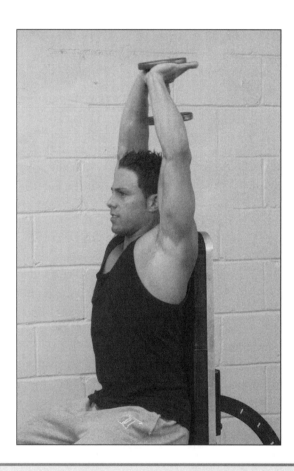
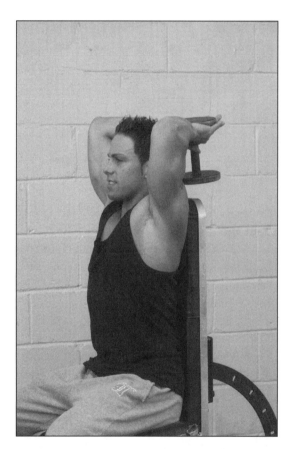

Mind Over Muscle Re-MIND-er:

Boost your energy levels during your workout by visualizing a time when you were feeling energized—a time when nothing could stop you if you didn't want to be stopped. It doesn't have to be a workout session; it could be a party, a special date, or just a time when everything was going well. Visualize the event and remember exactly how you felt. Doing so should stimulate your nervous system and heighten your energy level to new peaks. Also, tap into your emotions. Make yourself happy and excited during your workout; think about how good you look and feel. If you're angry, channel your anger at your weights, not yourself.

Overhead Rope Triceps Extension

PRIMARY TARGET MUSCLES: Triceps

NOTES: This exercise hits all three triceps heads along their full length, giving them an incredible workout. Because you'll be standing with the cable trying to pull you backward off your feet, it's absolutely crucial to maintain a proper stance throughout the exercise, with a staggered stance and slight forward bend at the hips. Otherwise you risk injury to your back.

EXECUTION AND FORM

Step 1: With the rope attachment connected to a low-pulley cable, stand with your back facing the pulley machine and take hold of the rope behind your head using a neutral grip with palms facing each other. The pinky side of your fists should be facing up at the rope ends and against the stops.

Step 2: Stand with your feet staggered, shoulder width apart and one foot about 6 inches in front of the other. Bend your knees slightly to reduce stress on the lower back.

Step 3: Your elbows should be next to your ears and pointed at the ceiling.

The forearms are bent at a 90-degree angle to the upper arms.

Step 4: Contract your abs to bend forward slightly at the hips and, with the elbows locked in place, contract the triceps isometrically to focus on their movement.

Step 5: With your concentration on the triceps, contract them and extend your forearms until they form a straight line with your upper arms. Avoid locking out the elbows. Though your hands may have been touching while behind your head, they will separate as you draw them upward.

Step 6: Slowly lower the forearms to the starting position. Remember not to move your upper arms and keep your elbows stationary next to your ears.

Step 7: At the bottom of the movement, when your arms are bent at 90 degrees, do not stop. Instead, contract the triceps for the next extension. Make the transition between reps a smooth one with fluid motion.

Overhead Rope Triceps Extension

SECONDARY TARGET MUSCLES: **Shoulders**

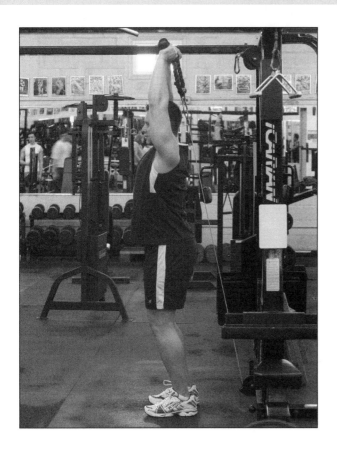
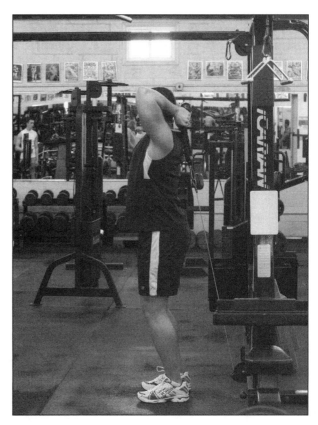

Mind Over Muscle Re-MIND-er:

In your training journal or on a whiteboard or chalkboard, draw a small circle for every set you're planning to do. Every time you finish a set, cross out or blacken in one of those circles. Let the sense of accomplishment you get from seeing what you've already done motivate you to finish the sets.

Dumbbell Triceps Kickback

PRIMARY TARGET MUSCLES: Triceps

NOTES: This is a great isolation exercise if you settle for using lighter weights and just concentrate on using good form. This exercise will provide you with a killer contraction at the top of the movement. Hold that contraction for a second or two in order to really fry those triceps.

EXECUTION AND FORM

Step 1: With this exercise, you will be training one arm at a time. Starting with the right triceps, lean down on a flat bench and place your left knee and your left hand on the bench for support. Your right leg will remain in a semi-straight position, with the foot flat on the floor. Maintain a flat back throughout the exercise.

Step 2: Pick up a dumbbell with one hand, making sure that the weight is light enough to maintain proper form throughout the exercise. Hold the weight at your side in a neutral wrist position, with the palm facing the bench.

Step 3: In the bent-over position, place the upper arm of your working hand tight against the right side of your body and parallel to your body. Make sure your lower arm is free to move.

Step 4: Begin the exercise with your elbow bent at a 90-degree angle. Concentrate on your triceps and flex it tightly prior to beginning the extension. With your mind fully on the triceps, contract the muscles and extend the lower arm back until it is at full extension and forms a nearly straight line with the upper arm.

Step 5: Make sure that you keep the upper arm pressed against the right side of the body during the exercise and that your elbow does not move.

Step 6: Once the arm reaches full extension, contract the triceps as hard as possible. Make sure to avoid hyperextension of the elbow.

Step 7: Slowly lower the forearm back to the 90-degree angle position you started in.

Dumbbell Triceps Kickback

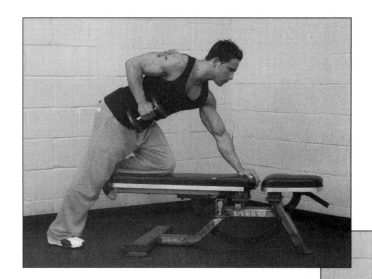

Mind Over Muscle Re-MIND-er:

To help you get in tune with your muscles and the movements of an exercise, set a new goal for each workout session to perfect a new part of the exercise. One week you may focus on keeping that elbow locked in place throughout the set. The next week you'll focus on squeezing the triceps at the top of the movement. This helps focus your concentration and programs your mind and body for correct performance. Eventually, your mind and muscles will automatically remember how to do the movement perfectly without having to consciously think about it.

Pulley Triceps Kickback

PRIMARY TARGET MUSCLES: **Outer Triceps**

NOTES: This is a variation of the dumbbell triceps kickback. Functionally, the main difference is that your hand will be in a supine position rather than a neutral position, allowing the movement to target the outer head of the triceps.

EXECUTION AND FORM

Step 1: With this exercise, you will be training one arm at a time. Stand in a staggered stance with a slight bend in the knees and facing the pulley. Bend at the hips and support your weight with the non-working hand by placing it on the pulley system's support handle.

Step 2: With a stirrup handle attachment on the low pulley cable, take the handle in a supinated grip (palm faces forward; your thumb points away from your body) with your palm facing forward.

Step 3: In the bent-over position, place the upper arm of your working hand tight against the right side of your body and parallel to the floor. Make sure your lower arm is free to move.

Step 4: Begin the exercise with your elbow bent at a 90-degree angle. Concentrate on your triceps and flex it tightly prior to beginning the extension. With your mind fully on the triceps, contract the muscles and extend the lower arm back until it is at full extension and forms a nearly straight line with the upper arm.

Step 5: Make sure that you keep the upper arm pressed against the right side of the body during the exercise and that your elbow does not move.

Step 6: Once the arm reaches full extension, contract the triceps as hard as possible. Make sure to avoid hyperextension of the elbow.

Step 7: Slowly lower the forearm back to the 90-degree angle position you started in.

Pulley Triceps Kickback

SECONDARY TARGET MUSCLES: Inner Triceps

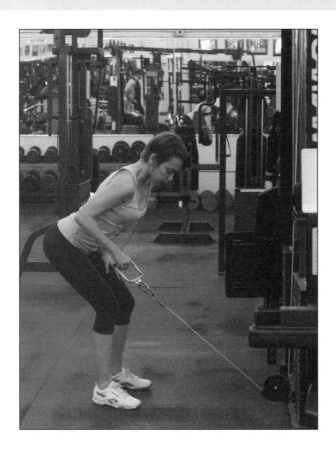
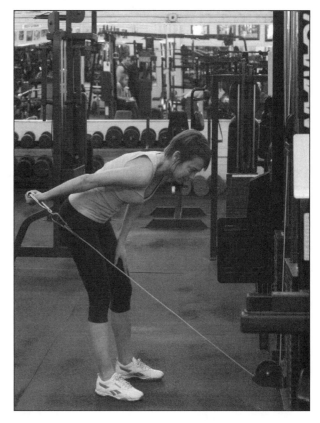

Mind Over Muscle Re-MIND-er:

To increase the mind-to-muscle connection and increase the "pump" a muscle gets from an exercise, practice the Flushing technique from time to time. When you've done the last rep you can do for a particular set, start another rep but stop several inches into the exercise. Hold the contraction at this point and let the muscle flush with blood. You'll feel an intense burn in the muscle.

Triceps Pushdown

PRIMARY TARGET MUSCLES: Triceps

> **NOTES:** This exercise is often performed incorrectly. Some common mistakes include the following:
> - Too much bending at the hips, which incorporates chest muscle activity. Stay as straight as possible with a very slight bend to prevent lower back injury.
> - Bending over far enough that the cable is forced to go past one side of the head. This causes an imbalance of resistance. Keep your body as straight as possible with the cable at the center of your body.
> - Allowing the arms to come up during the negative portion of the exercise. Keep the upper arms locked at the sides of the body until the end of the exercise. Only the forearms should move.
>
> You can use a V-shaped bar attachment or a rope attachment for this exercise. Choose the attachment that provides the more comfortable grip.

EXECUTION AND FORM

Step 1: Stand in front of the cable and take hold of the V-bar or rope. Pull it down by bringing your elbows to the sides of your body and lock them there.

Step 2: Position your feet shoulder width apart with your feet pointing straight ahead. Slightly bend your knees and keep your torso upright throughout the movement. Keep your head pointing straight ahead and avoid looking down; otherwise you will tend to bend over.

Step 3: Holding the bar with your arms with forearms perpendicular to the upper arms, and elbows locked in place at your sides, begin by isometrically contracting the triceps muscles before moving the bar down.

Step 4: Contract the triceps and push the bar down while keeping your elbows pinned to your sides.

Step 5: Press down until you have reached full extension. Avoid locking the elbow joint out hard. Squeeze the triceps muscles as hard as you possibly can. Focus on squeezing the triceps muscles hard, not the elbow joint.

Step 6: When you've reached the bottom position, squeeze the triceps muscles. Allow the bar to rise in a controlled manner while maintaining your posture and arms at the sides.

Step 7: Let the bar or rope come up so that your forearms are slightly higher than parallel to the floor. Without resting begin pushing down to the bottom position again. Stay focused on the triceps.

Triceps Pushdown

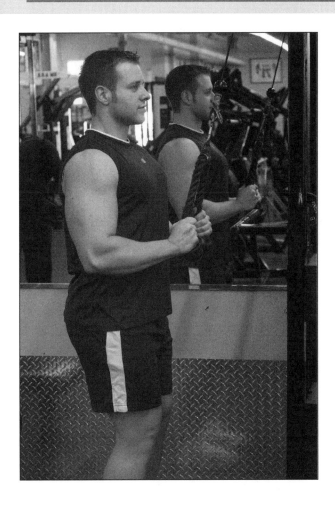

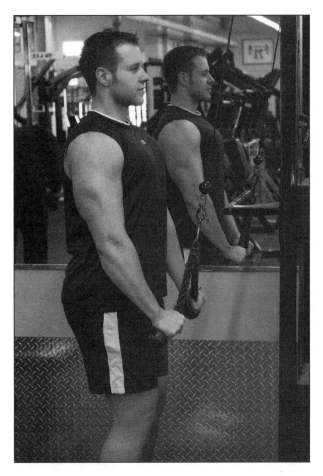

Mind Over Muscle Re-**MIND**-er:

The mind tends to wander, but you have to get it focused to get in the zone and stay there for the duration of your workout. State out loud to yourself what you plan to do before you begin an exercise. Be simple and realistic. Even if you don't reach your intended number of reps, saying what you want to do is a surefire way to pull your focus back to the task at hand. Between sets, think about how you work harder and are more disciplined than anyone else around you.

Machine Triceps Extension

PRIMARY TARGET MUSCLES: Triceps (middle and inner heads)

NOTES: This exercise has the advantage of making it easy to keep proper form no matter how much weight is being used. The machine also isolates the triceps very thoroughly. If you're not familiar with how the triceps should feel during an exercise, the triceps machine is a good way to start.

EXECUTION AND FORM

Step 1: Select a weight and sit in the machine's seat with your arms positioned overhead.

Step 2: Bend your arms at the elbow and grab the bar or rope with both hands. Your upper arms will now be at a 90-degree angle, as your forearms are angled backwards.

Step 3: Contract your triceps isometrically and draw your concentration into the muscles. Tighten your abs and begin to force the bar or rope up to full extension, where your forearms are above your upper arms. Throughout the movement, try to keep your elbows pinched closer to your head. If the elbows float away, you will not be isolating your triceps.

Step 4: When you reach the fully extended position, in which you should maintain a slight bend in the elbows to maintain tension, squeeze the triceps hard.

Step 5: Return to the starting position while resisting the weight along the way.

Step 6: Without any rest and avoiding the use of momentum, squeeze the triceps and press the weight back up to the top position. Keep your elbows locked in place and your body in correct alignment.

Machine Triceps Extension

SECONDARY TARGET MUSCLES: **Triceps (outer head)**

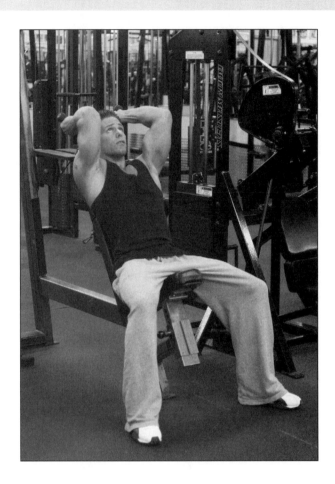

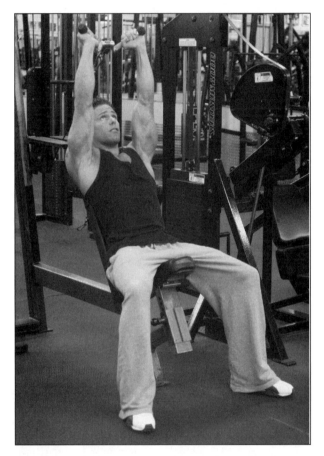

Mind Over Muscle Re-**MIND**-er:

Don't forget to visualize every rep. In addition to feeling the muscle work, you have to envision the effects of that movement. See the muscle pull at the same time you feel it and your body will do what it's supposed to. When your muscles are searing with pain, make someone else hurt. To get your last few reps in, tell yourself that the burning you think you feel actually belongs to the person next to you and, suddenly, you don't feel a thing.

Isometric Bicep Curl and Triceps Extension

PRIMARY TARGET MUSCLES: **Biceps or Triceps**

> **NOTES:** If you are traveling or don't have access to weights, curls and extensions can be done with isometric resistance. The biceps and triceps of opposite arms resist each other instead of using weights. The Two-Step Rep is actually more of a Three-Step rep with three seconds to extend the arm and three seconds to curl the arm.

EXECUTION AND FORM

Step 1: Clasp your hands together in front of you with an arm-wrestling like grip. Put your elbows at your sides and lower your hands together until your arms are as extended as possible without moving your elbows.

Step 2: With the hand that has the palm-up grip, perform a bicep curl and resist the movement with the opposite hand. The resisting hand should primarily be using the triceps.

Step 3: Once you've reached the full contraction press down with the triceps arm and resist with your curling arm. At the bottom switch hands and repeat.

Mind Over Muscle Re-**MIND**-er:

To help you get in tune with your muscles and the movements of an exercise, set a new goal for each workout session to perfect a new part of the exercise. One week you may focus on keeping that elbow locked in place throughout the set. The next week you'll focus on squeezing the triceps at the top of the movement. This helps focus your concentration and programs your mind and body for correct performance. Eventually, your mind and muscles will automatically remember how to do the movement perfectly without having to consciously think about it. Keep your focus on the biceps or triceps, not the elbow.

Isometric Bicep Curl and Triceps Extension

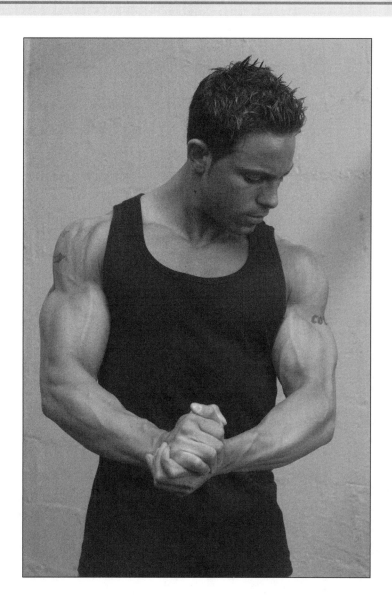

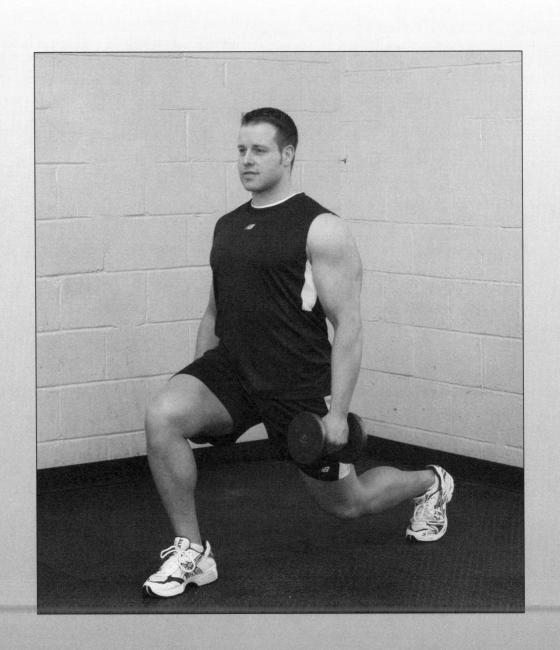

Chapter 8:

Leg and Abdominal Exercises

Legs

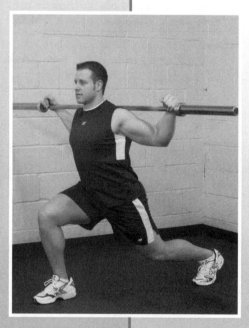

- Barbell Squat
- Dumbbell Squat
- Bodyweight Squat
- Barbell Lunge
- Dumbbell Lunge
- Leg Press
- Wide Stance Leg Press
- Leg Extension
- Standing Leg Curl
- Lying Leg Curl
- Calf Press
- Dumbbell Calf Raise
- Standing Calf Raise Machine
- Seated Calf Raise

Barbell Squat

PRIMARY TARGET MUSCLES: Quadriceps

NOTES: Squatting with a barbell typically allows you to use heavier weights because the weight is supported by your entire body rather than trying to hold onto it with just your hands. The wide stance version emphasizes the inside of the thighs more than the outside muscles.

EXECUTION AND FORM

Step 1: Place a bar on either a squat safety rack or in a power cage, making sure you have the safety bars set about even with your hips when you are standing up. In this position, the safety bars will keep you from getting crushed if you lose control on the bottom of the movement.

Step 2: Align your body from the bottom up by first taking a shoulder width stance with feet pointed straight ahead.
- **WIDE STANCE VERSION:** Stand with your feet about hip-width apart and point your toes out slightly.

Step 3: Slightly bend your knees and avoid locking them during this exercise. Contract your abdominal muscles to help support and sustain your posture during the exercise. Stick your chest out and simultaneously bring your shoulder blades back, keeping them there throughout the movement.

Step 4: Keep your head level at all times, making sure your head or your eyes do not drop down, or excessively wander upward. This is an easy way to lose your balance and fall. It is preferable to look slightly above level rather than below because looking below level can greatly affect your equilibrium and jeopardize your safety.

Step 5: If you feel unstable, you may put small weight plates under each heel.

Step 6: Duck under the bar and with a shoulder width overhand grip, use your shoulders to unrack the barbell. Readjust your alignment in the full upright position before you continue.

Step 7: Contract your glutes and flex your thighs, then descend by bending your knees. Remember to keep your back straight. Your shins should be in a vertical line throughout the move.

Step 8: As you are squatting, it is very important that your knees never go forward beyond your toes. This puts way too much pressure on the knees and can seriously damage them. If you're having trouble with that, mimic the motion and alignment of sitting in a chair. Make sure you keep your back as straight as possible. This motion will naturally help you keep proper form.

Step 9: Don't let your thighs go below parallel, as you could injure your lower back or push the knees past your toes, once again leading to injury.

Step 10: As you reach parallel or just above it, exhale and press off your feet, distributing the weight through the heels while pressing upward. Concentrate on keeping and holding proper alignment throughout the movement. Feel your thigh and glute muscles contract through the ascent.

Step 11: At the top, do not lock out your knees since it will put too much stress on the joint. If at any time during the movement you should feel or

Barbell Squat

SECONDARY TARGET MUSCLES: Hamstrings, Gluteals, Calves

notice yourself getting sloppy or not retaining the proper alignment, stop immediately! Never jeopardize your safety with bad form.

Step 12: When you've done your desired amount of reps, rack the barbell at the top of your final squat.

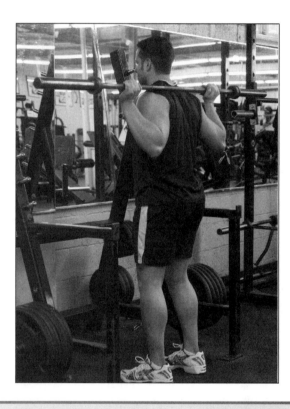

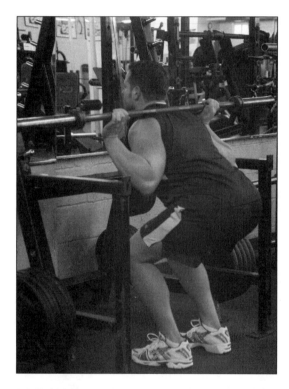

Mind Over Muscle Re-**MIND**-er:

Squats, once you've become accustomed to using correct form and when done safely in a squat safety rack, in a power cage, or on a Smith Machine, are a good exercise in which to challenge yourself. Your legs are immensely powerful and can often do more than you think. Challenge yourself to lift heavier, do more reps, or rest less between sets and see what you can handle when you put your full concentration and confidence into an exercise. Don't be afraid to challenge yourself—just be safe when doing so. You must learn to know your limits. There is a difference between a safe challenge and a stupid one. It's always a great idea to have a qualified person spot you whenever you choose to take that next challenge step. The Full Body Tension Technique is ideal for this exercise.

Dumbbell Squat

PRIMARY TARGET MUSCLES: Quadriceps

NOTES: One of the best exercises you can do to build strong, ripped legs is the squat. Squats also provide beneficial results to the whole body because several body muscles synergistically join forces to execute the lift. It incorporates virtually all the body's major muscle groups in one way or another. Note that performing the exercise with dumbbells puts excessive stress on the lower back if you don't contract your glutes and keep them under tight tension. The wide stance version emphasizes the inside of the thighs more than the outside muscles. When you work up to particularly heavy dumbbells, use wrist straps to help maintain your grip throughout the set.

EXECUTION AND FORM

Step 1: Hold a dumbbell in each hand with arms extended down and palms facing your body.

Step 2: Align your body from the bottom up by first taking a stance with feet about shoulder-width apart and angle your toes out slightly.

Step 3: Slightly bend your knees and avoid locking them during this exercise. Contract your abdominal muscles to help support and sustain your posture during the exercise. Stick your chest out and simultaneously bring your shoulder blades back, keeping them there throughout the movement.

Step 4: Keep your head level at all times, making sure your head or your eyes do not drop down, or excessively wander upward. This is an easy way to lose your balance and fall. It is preferable to look slightly above

level rather than below because looking below level can greatly affect your equilibrium and jeopardize your safety.

Step 5: If you feel unstable, you may put small weight plates under each heel.

Step 6: Contract your glutes and flex your thighs, then descend by bending your knees. Remember to keep your back straight. Your shins should be in a vertical line throughout the move.

Step 7: As you are squatting, it is very important that your knees never go forward beyond your toes. This puts way too much pressure on the knees and can seriously damage them. If you're having trouble with that, mimic the motion and alignment of sitting in a chair. Make sure you keep your back as straight as possible. This

motion will naturally help you keep proper form.

Step 8: Don't let your thighs go below parallel, as you could injure your lower back or push the knees past your toes, which could lead to injury.

Step 9: As you reach parallel or just above it, exhale and press off your feet, distributing the weight through the heels while pressing upward. Concentrate on keeping and holding proper alignment throughout the movement. Feel your thigh and glute muscles contract through the ascent.

Step 10: At the top, do not lock out your knees since it will put too much stress on the joint. If at any time during the movement you notice yourself getting sloppy or not retaining the proper alignment, stop immediately! Never jeopardize your safety with bad form.

Dumbbell Squat

SECONDARY TARGET MUSCLES: Hamstrings, Gluteals, Calves

Step 11: When you've done your desired amount of reps, simply squat down once again and place the dumbbells on the floor or place them back on the dumbbell rack. Never bend over to either pick up or place the dumbbells down. Doing this can injure your lower back.

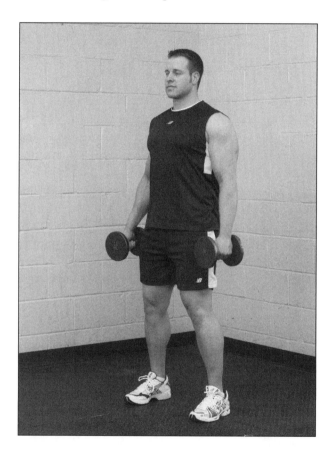

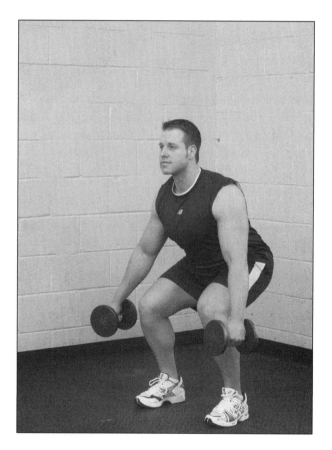

Mind Over Muscle Re-**MIND**-er:

Before picking up the dumbbells at the start of a set, assume your working stance and use the Full Body Tension Technique. Doing so prepares your body for action and bearing the weight. Maintain the tension as you pick up the dumbbells and tense with them for a moment before beginning the set. Just before starting the first rep, switch your attention and tensing to the quads or whatever muscle group is being worked.

Bodyweight Squat

PRIMARY TARGET MUSCLES: **Thighs**

NOTES: This exercise can be done anywhere. Because you're not using any extra weight, bodyweight squats require vastly more repetitions to peak the muscles for growth. Done at a quick pace, it can be a good cardiovascular exercise as well as a strength builder.

EXECUTION AND FORM

Step 1: Stand erect with your feet shoulder width apart and your knees slightly bent. You can either point your toes straight ahead or angle your toes slightly outward. Your arms are hanging straight at your sides.

Step 2: Keep your head straight and looking forward throughout the exercise.

Step 3: Contract your thigh muscles and glutes in a tight, isometric squeeze before you begin.

Step 4: Bend your knees and push your butt back as you lower it toward the ground. Keep your back straight or with a slight arch in the lower back. On the descent you can raise your arms out in front of you to act as a counter balance and keep you from falling backward.

Step 5: Stop the descent when your thighs are parallel to the ground or as far as you can while maintaining your balance and keeping your back straight.

Step 6: Hold the bottom position in a tight contraction. Give your glutes an extra squeeze to help you on your way back up. Lower your arms as you come up so you don't overstress the upper back and pull it out of alignment.

ADVANCED EXERCISERS: Instead of stopping with thighs at parallel, lift the heels off the ground and touch your butt to them. Again, squeeze the glutes before you begin the ascent as this will stabilize and strengthen your form. This method can also be done one leg at a time with the non-working leg stretched out in front of you. If you attempt this exercise, keep your heel on the ground or elevated on a small weight plate.

Bodyweight Squat

SECONDARY TARGET MUSCLES: Hamstrings, Gluteals

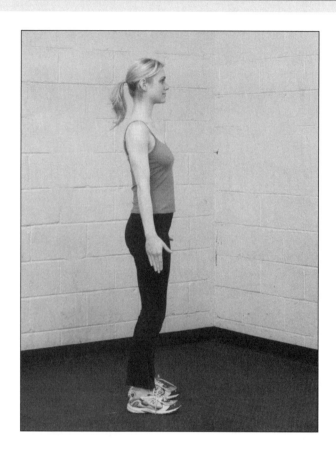

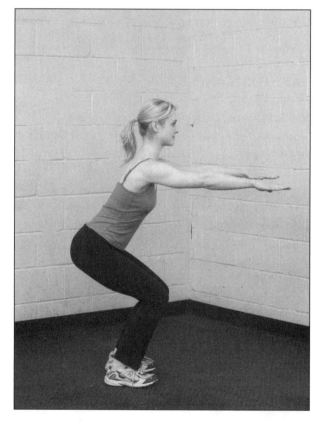

Mind Over Muscle Re-**MIND**-er:

When the burn sets in on high-rep sets and you think you're about to collapse, hand that pain to somebody else. Tell yourself that pain belongs to the person next to you and that you don't really feel any pain at all. Believe it and the pain will fade away as you finish your set. You might also want to try the Flushing technique with this exercise from time to time. It is a great way to really bring in lots of beneficial blood to the areas of the legs, and will really challenge those leg muscles.

Barbell Lunge

PRIMARY TARGET MUSCLES: **Thighs, Gluteals, Hamstrings**

NOTES: Because only one leg is used at a time, lunges require a balancing act. In order to maintain balance, the body recruits as many auxiliary fibers as possible. This means more muscle stimulation per repetition. In addition, lunges can stimulate the hamstring muscles or the quadriceps muscles by varying how far away you place your foot. If you step forward with your foot closer to your body, you will primarily stimulate the quadriceps. If you step forward with your foot farther away, you will primarily stimulate the hamstrings. Warning: In no case, as you'll see in the exercise description, should your knee go past your toes. The barbell variation places more stress on the lower back, so remember to keep your back straight and vertical.

EXECUTION AND FORM

Step 1: Place a relatively light barbell across your shoulders, as if you were doing a squat.

Step 2: Align your body from the bottom up, taking a stance with the feet together and toes pointing straight ahead. Keep your knees slightly bent to avoid any stress from locking the knee joint. Slightly contract the abdominal muscles.

Step 3: Stick the chest out while simultaneously bringing the shoulder blades back, keeping them there throughout the movement. Keep your head level at all times, making sure your head or your eyes do not drop down or excessively wander upward.

Step 4: Step forward with your right foot. Bend at the knees, making sure you descend slowly and in control and that your right knee does not go past your toes. As your left knee bends and your hips are lowering, lower yourself only until your left knee is about two inches from the ground and then stop.

Step 5: Reverse the movement by pushing through the heel of your right foot only. You may naturally want to use the left knee to assist in pushing back up, but do not let this happen. The objective is to fully isolate the right leg muscles and use the left leg only as a balancing tool, sort of like the rudder on a boat. Remember to keep your focus on

the contraction of your right thigh muscle throughout the exercise.

Step 6: Make sure you do not use momentum as you push off with the right leg to return. This will totally inhibit the stimulation of the leg muscles.

Step 7: Return to the start position but do not rest. Switch legs and repeat the same movement, making sure to maintain the alignment and posture throughout the movement. Once you've lunged with both legs, congratulations: you've completed one repetition.

Barbell Lunge

SECONDARY TARGET MUSCLES: **Calves**

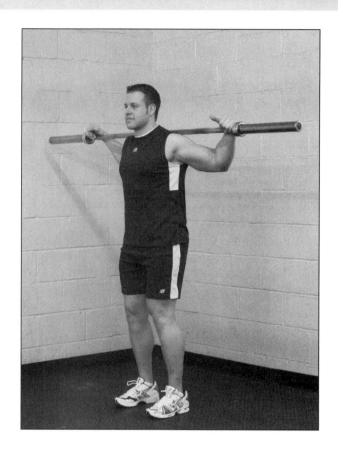

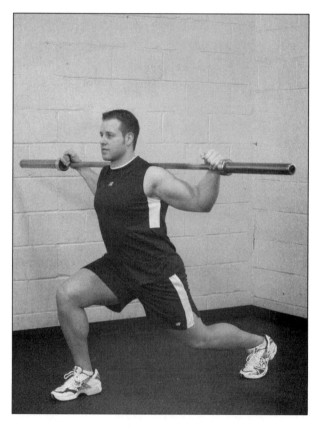

Mind Over Muscle Re-**MIND**-er:

Some people think that you have to be loose and springy to avoid injury on an exercise like the lunge. Actually, tensing your leg muscles in this exercise stabilizes your joints and absorbs the impact to reduce the risk of injury. It's like a seatbelt in a car accident: a snug one will keep you tight against the seatback and limits whiplash, while a loose one lets your body gain forward momentum before jolting you to a stop. Now you know why so many guys use lifting belts during their workouts. Just like a tight seatbelt, it makes them feel more secure.

191

Dumbbell Lunge

PRIMARY TARGET MUSCLES: Thighs, Gluteals, Hamstrings

> **NOTES:** Generally, it's easier to keep your balance with dumbbell lunges than with the barbell version. However, dumbbells are harder to go heavy with because it's dependent on your grip strength. Just like barbell lunges, dumbbell lunges require a balancing act that causes the body to recruit as many auxiliary fibers as possible and stimulate more muscle growth. Remember, if you step forward with your foot closer to your body, you will primarily stimulate the quadriceps, but you will primarily stimulate the hamstrings if you step forward with your foot farther away.

EXECUTION AND FORM

Step 1: Hold a dumbbell in each hand with arms extended down and palms facing your body.

Step 2: Align your body from the bottom up, taking a stance with the feet together and toes pointing straight ahead. Keep your knees slightly bent to avoid any stress from locking the knee joint. Slightly contract the abdominal muscles.

Step 3: Stick the chest out while simultaneously bringing the shoulder blades back, keeping them there throughout the movement. Keep your head level at all times, making sure your head or your eyes do not drop down or excessively wander upward.

Step 4: Step forward with your right foot. Bend at the knees, making sure you descend slowly and in control and that your right knee does not go past your toes. As your left knee bends and your hips are lowering, lower yourself only until your left knee is about two inches from the ground and then stop.

Step 5: Reverse the movement by pushing off the right foot only. You may naturally want to use the left knee to assist in pushing back up, but do not let this happen. The objective is to fully isolate the right leg muscles and use the left leg only as a balancing tool, sort of like the rudder on a boat. Remember to keep your focus on the contraction of

your right thigh muscle throughout the exercise.

Step 6: Make sure you do not use momentum as you push off with the right leg to return. This will totally inhibit the stimulation of the leg muscles.

Step 7: Return to the start position but do not rest. Switch legs and repeat the same movement, making sure to maintain the alignment and posture throughout the movement. Once you've lunged with both legs, you've completed one repetition.

Dumbbell Lunge

SECONDARY TARGET MUSCLES: Calves

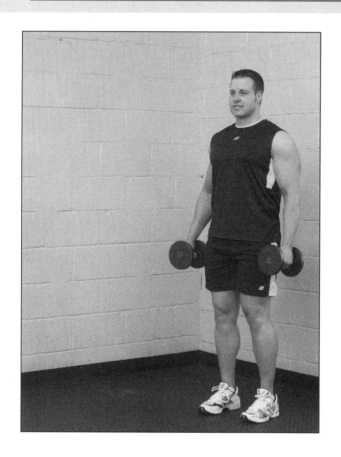

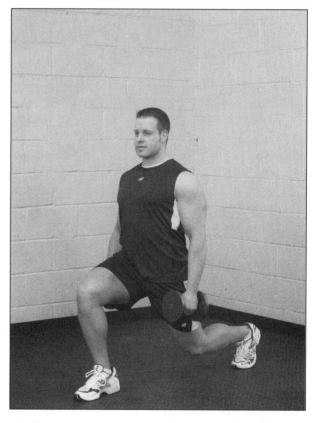

Mind Over Muscle Re-**MIND**-er:

Don't forget your back in an exercise like lunges. Although your thigh, hamstrings, and glutes are involved primarily, forgetting about your back can cause it to come out of alignment and result in injury. Without taking your concentration off the main muscles, try to develop an awareness of your back. Hey, if you're stumped by how to do that, think of it this way: it will keep you coming "back" to the gym!

Leg Press

PRIMARY TARGET MUSCLES: Thighs

NOTES: This exercise can be used in place of the traditional barbell squat for people that suffer from lower back pain, as a rehabilitation exercise, or to supplement your leg routine. You can typically handle more weight on a leg press than with a squat because the lower back is taken out of the equation.

EXECUTION AND FORM

Step 1: Sit on the machine with your back on the padded support and align your feet evenly on the platform about hip width apart.

Step 2: This particular foot placement will zone in on quadriceps of your front thigh. Placing your feet higher on the platform will slightly lessen the effects on the quadriceps, but will minimize the stress on the knee. The lower foot placement on the platform will increase the quadriceps contraction but puts more stress on the knee. If you do go lower on the platform please do not sacrifice your safety for quantity.

Step 3: Make sure that your back and head are kept flush against the back pad and that you are seated securely in the seat. Focus on your quads and contract them.

Step 4: Contract the quads and press the platform away. When your legs are fully extended, take hold of the release lever handles and disengage the lock pins. Immediately take hold of the secured handles, which are usually located to the sides of you. If the handles are placed in an awkward position, you can also take hold of the seat edge. This can take some stress off the lower back.

Step 5: With the feet spaced evenly apart and flat upon the platform, slowly lower the platform toward you while concentrating on the quads. Do not grip the handles too tightly.

Step 6: Let the sled and platform come down to a point just before your thighs would touch your chest or low enough where your back is not lifted off of the seat rest.

Step 7: When you have reached the bottom portion of the exercise, return back to the starting position by slowly pushing the platform evenly with both feet. Do not lock your knees on the extension! This could injure them and will take the resistance off the quads, distributing it directly to the knee joints.

Leg Press

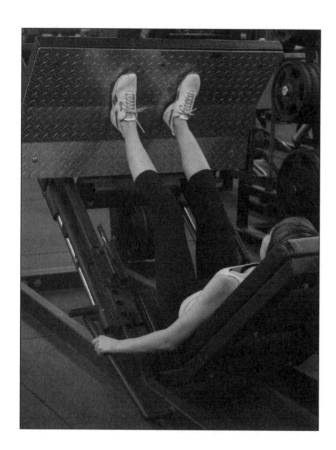

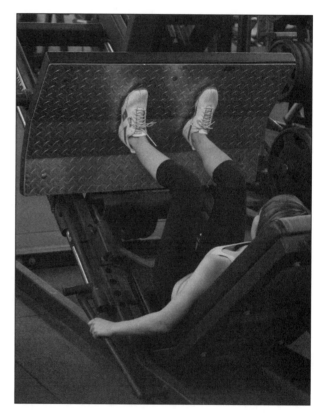

Mind Over Muscle Re-**MIND**-er:

Instead of pressing, imagine you are leaping away from the foot plate. Think Superman-type leaps that will take you to the top of a building in a single bound. It may sound like a simple thing, but merely changing the way you think about an exercise sends new signals to the muscles, which causes them to put new effort into the movement. Focus on keeping the weight evenly distributed throughout this exercise.

Wide Stance Leg Press

PRIMARY TARGET MUSCLES: **Thighs, Hamstrings, Hip Adductors**

NOTES: This exercise can be used in place of the traditional barbell squat for people who suffer from lower back pain, as a rehabilitation exercise, or to supplement your leg routine. The wide stance places more emphasis on the inner thighs and ham- strings.

EXECUTION AND FORM

Step 1: Sit on the machine with your back on the padded support and align your feet evenly on the platform a little more than shoulder width apart. If the platform is not wide enough for that, place your feet as far apart as possible without risking that they will slip off the sides of the platform while pressing.

Step 2: The height placement of your feet on the platform will zone in on different areas of the quadriceps. Placing your feet higher lessens the quad contraction and minimizes stress on the knee, while lower placement increases quad contraction but puts more stress on the knee. Use a higher foot placement here.

Step 3: Make sure that your back and head are kept flush against the back

pad and that you are seated securely in the seat. Focus on your quads and hamstrings and contract them.

Step 4: Contract the quads and press the platform away. When your legs are fully extended, take hold of the release lever handles and disengage the lock pins. Immediately take hold of the secured handles, which are usually located to the sides of you. If the handles are placed in an awkward position, you can also take hold of the seat edge. This can take some stress off the lower back.

Step 5: With the feet spaced evenly apart and flat upon the platform, slowly lower the platform toward you while concentrating on the quads. Do not grip the handles too tightly.

Step 6: Let the sled and platform come down to a point just before your thighs would touch your chest.

Step 7: When you have reached the bottom portion of the exercise, return back to the starting position by slowly pushing the platform evenly with both feet. Do not lock your knees on the extension! This could injure them and will take the resistance off the quads, distributing it directly to the knee joints.

Wide Stance Leg Press

SECONDARY TARGET MUSCLES: **Hamstrings, Gluteals**

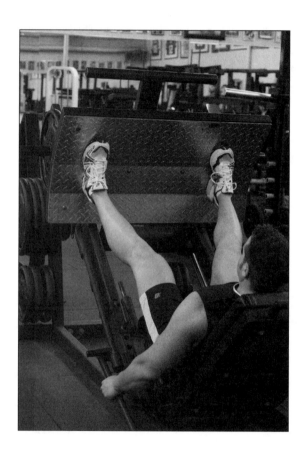 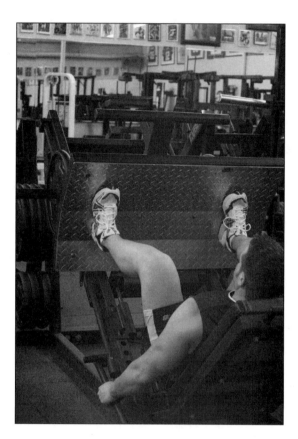

Mind Over Muscle Re-**MIND**-er:

To really get those leg muscles stimulated, make sure to keep the tension constant (using the Time Under Tension principle). In other words, try not to take breaks at the top or bottom of the movement. If you need a break, by all means, take it. If you know you can keep going and have the energy and power to do so, than keep that motion going. Keep it smooth and fluid throughout the duration of the exercise.

Leg Extension

PRIMARY TARGET MUSCLES: Quadriceps

NOTES: Extensions help strengthen the knee, which is a commonly injured area. It is recommended by most physical therapists as a good tool for knee rehabilitation. The key to the effectiveness and safety of this exercise is to choose a machine whose starting position allows your toes to be right in front of your knees and to focus on contracting the thigh muscle. Don't overdo the weights; focusing on lifting heavy weights will cause knee damage, especially if you are using a machine in which your toes start behind your knees. You can do this exercise one leg at a time or with both legs. Execution for the exercise is the same for both versions, though here I will use the two-leg version. If you're traveling or don't have access to weight machines, perform this exercise isometrically by using the leg biceps (hamstrings) to resist the quads.

EXECUTION AND FORM

Step 1: Seat yourself on the machine and position the back pad so that you are sitting totally upright.

Step 2: The back of your knees must be pressed flush against the front of the seat, which will help you avoid a potential knee injury. Doing this will give the needed support to your knees. You also want to make sure that the axis of the knees is in line with the machine axis, helping to set up the proper alignment of the knee and direct the maximum resistance to the quadriceps. Make sure the toes are in front of the knees and that the upper leg and lower leg create a 90-degree angle.

Step 3: Adjust the shin roller pad against the lowest point of the shin to help optimize the shin as a lever and the knee as the fulcrum. This will again help to direct the majority of the resistance to the thigh muscles.

Before you begin the exercise, grip the handles provided or grab the front of the seat on each side of your legs.

Step 4: Begin with your legs totally relaxed and your shins behind the roller pad positioned at the bottom. Isometrically contract the quad muscles and slowly begin to lift the weight by lifting the roller pad with the shins.

Step 5: As you extend your legs, stay in control by allowing the quad muscles to lift the weight. Do not use momentum or leverage. This is a very easy exercise to cheat on by using quick bursts of momentum at the bottom of the movement, or by leaning back and using leverage to lift the weight.

Step 6: As you reach the point of full extension, when your shins are extended in a nearly direct line with

your upper thigh, focus only on fully contracting the quad muscles. As long as you make a great effort to squeeze or contract the quad muscle fully at the top of full extension, you will be taking full advantage of the exercise.

Step 7: Make sure that once you get to the fully extended position of the exercise, you don't just let the leg drop, but slowly return back to the beginning of the movement in a controlled fashion. Feel the quads flex during the lowering motion.

Step 8: When you reach the bottom, do not rest. Slowly and smoothly begin the next extension. Always go through the full range of motion for these exercises to provide the maximum muscular development.

Leg Extension

SECONDARY TARGET MUSCLES: Calves

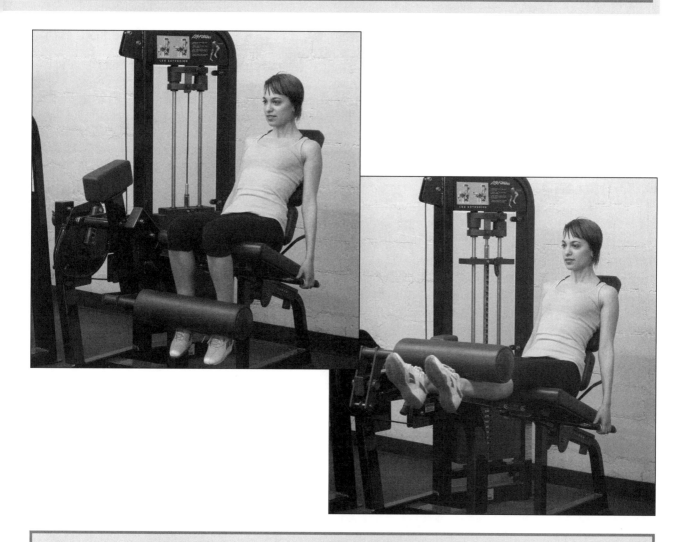

Mind Over Muscle Re-**MIND**-er:

Did you know you can make the muscle on one side of a joint stronger by flexing the muscle on the opposite side? When you're about two-thirds of the way through a set, pause in a rest position and contract the opposing muscle, such as the hamstrings for this exercise, for 10 seconds then maintain that hamstring tension as you complete the set. The hamstring tells the quad it can handle the load if the quad gets out of hand, so the quad has permission to recruit more muscle fibers and maximize its power.

Standing Leg Curl

PRIMARY TARGET MUSCLES: Hamstrings (leg biceps)

NOTES: The standing leg curl does more to isolate the hamstring muscles, reduce strain on the glutes and lower back, and focus on possible imbalances between the two legs than the lying leg curl does. Remember that form is more important than using heavy weight for leg curls. It is very easy to pull a hamstring if you are using heavy weights and trying to jerk them. This exercise can be done isometrically when you're traveling or when you can't get to a leg curl machine; just use your quads to resist the hamstrings.

EXECUTION AND FORM

Step 1: Stand next to the lever arm of the leg curl machine so that it is to the right of your leg. Hook your right heel under the roller pad attached to the lever arm. The type of machine you have access to will either allow you to kneel upon the knee rest with your left leg or stand with your left leg on a platform, which will keep your body elevated for your right leg to clear the platform when performing the exercise movement.

Step 2: Lock your pelvis into place by contracting your abdominal muscles.

Step 3: Focus your concentration on the hamstring muscles and flex them.

Step 4: Relax your upper body (Allowing your body to stay tense during the exercise will only negatively affect hamstring stimula-tion.) If you like, you can hold on to the set of handles, which are usually supplied. Just make sure you do so with a very light grip. Squeezing too hard can change the focus of resis-tance in the hamstring muscles, causing this exercise to be less bene-ficial. Holding too tight can also cause leverage to do the work for you instead of working the muscle.

Step 5: As you begin the movement, contract the hamstrings of your working leg before actually moving, as this will help to focus the resis-tance on the hamstring muscles, which will better stimulate those muscles.

Step 6: Drive your heel to your butt, while flexing your foot toward your knees. It will be the same whether sitting or lying down. This is very important; it helps to better isolate the hamstring muscles.

Step 7: When you reach your butt, or get as close as you can to it, squeeze the hamstring hard. This will increase the intensity of the exercise and better stimulate the hamstring muscles.

Step 8: As you return to the starting position, do so with a slow, controlled movement. When you reach the start-ing position, without rest, slowly and smoothly change directions, moving upward once again. Following these guidelines will ensure your safety and greater results.

Step 9: When you finish a set with one leg, immediately get your sec-ond leg into position and do a set with that leg.

Standing Leg Curl

SECONDARY TARGET MUSCLES: **Gluteals, Lower Back**

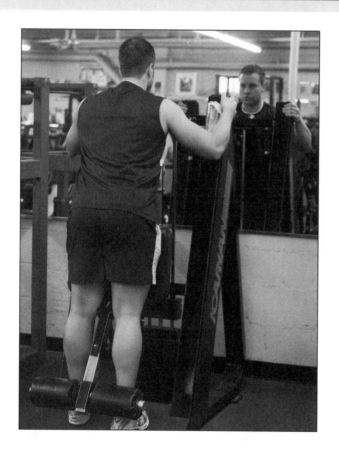

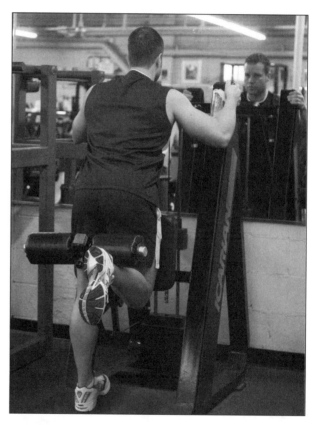

Mind Over Muscle Re-**MIND**-er:

Make sure you pay as much attention to the eccentric motion, or lowering of the weight, in the leg curl as you do to the concentric motion, or lifting part. The eccentric portion does just as much to stimulate muscle growth, and there is some indication that it actually does more to stimulate growth than the lifting portion. Always make sure not to lower the weight too quickly. Use a controlled and strict manner instead to work the muscle during both phases of the rep: lifting and lowering. This is a great exercise for the Flushing technique.

Lying Leg Curl

PRIMARY TARGET MUSCLES: Hamstrings

NOTES: It is very easy to pull a hamstring if you are using heavy weights and trying to jerk them so be careful not to use momentum. Leg curls are the leg equivalent of a barbell curl. The lying leg curl can be done one leg at a time or both legs at the same time.

EXECUTION AND FORM

Step 1: Position yourself on the machine and align your body by placing the backs of your ankles on the underside of the lifting pad with your feet at right angles to your shins.

Step 2: Lock your pelvis into place by contracting your abdominal muscles.

Step 3: Focus your concentration on the hamstring muscles and flex them.

Step 4: Relax your upper body. Allowing your body to stay tense during the exercise will only negatively affect hamstring stimulation. If you like, you can hold on to the set of handles, which are usually supplied. Just make sure you do so with a very light grip. Squeezing too

hard can change the focus of resistance in the hamstring muscles, causing this exercise to be less beneficial. Holding too tight can also cause leverage to do the work for you instead of working the muscle.

Step 5: As you begin the movement, contract the hamstrings before actually moving to help focus the resistance on the hamstring muscles, which will better stimulate those muscles.

Step 6: Drive your heels to your butt while flexing your feet toward your knees. Flexing your feet is very important, because it helps to better isolate the hamstring muscles.

Step 7: When you reach your butt, or as close as you can get to it, squeeze the hamstrings hard. This will

increase the intensity of the exercise and better stimulate the hamstring muscles.

Step 8: As you return to the starting position, do so with a slow, controlled movement that resists the weight. When you reach the starting position, without rest, slowly and smoothly change directions, moving upward once again. Following these guidelines will ensure your safety and greater results.

ONE-LEGGED CURLS: When you finish a set with one leg, immediately get your second leg into position and do a set with that leg.

Lying Leg Curl

SECONDARY TARGET MUSCLES: Gluteals, Lower Back

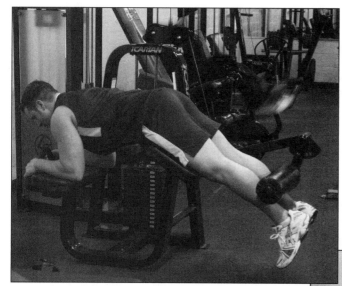

Mind Over Muscle Re-MIND-er:

Concentrate on squeezing your leg biceps. Envision how they form a ball as they pull up that lower leg. Visualize that the goal of the movement is to form that ball of muscle, not to lift the weight. Picture your hamstring muscles like they're nothing more than huge biceps muscles. It's not that much of a "stretch," actually. They work very similarly.

Calf Press

PRIMARY TARGET MUSCLES: **Calves (outer head)**

NOTES: This exercise is an excellent alternative to standing calf raises for people with lower back injuries. You can perform this with one leg or both legs at a time. Execution is the same for both versions.

EXECUTION AND FORM

Step 1: Sit down at the machine and place your feet on the foot plate of the machine about three to five inches apart.

Step 2: Position your feet on the foot plate so only the upper edge of your foot rests on it and the other half hangs off. Take hold of the handles, which are usually located to the sides of the machine.

Step 3: Keep the legs straight during the exercise with your knees slightly bent. Contract your calf muscles and feel where they are. Stay focused on the calves throughout the exercise.

Step 4: Maintaining your form, press your toes forward as far as you can and hold for two seconds. Focus on contracting the calf muscles.

Step 5: Slowly relax your calves, letting the toes and the foot plate come back toward you in a controlled manner.

Calf Press

SECONDARY TARGET MUSCLES: **Calves (inner head)**

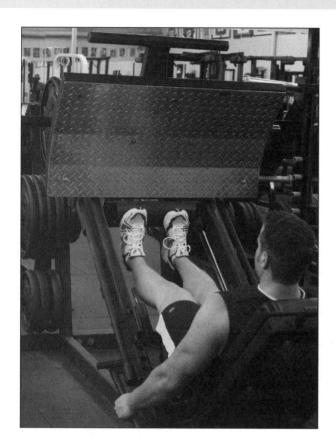
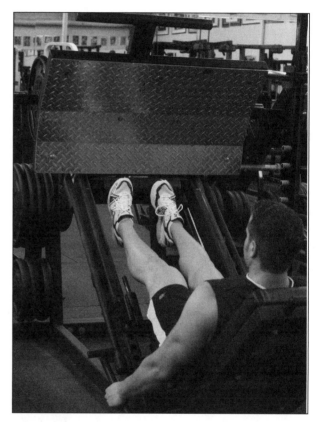

Mind Over Muscle Re-**MIND**-er:

The day you are most likely to injure yourself during a workout is the day you go to the gym distracted by other things. When you're thinking about work, or home, or the bills, or a conversation that went awry, your mind is not on the workout, keeping proper form, or tensing stabilizing muscles. Not focusing on those things leads to injury. Make sure you take time before each workout to calm your mind and put everything else out of your thoughts. If you can't, it might be safer to go take care of the things you're thinking about before you begin lifting.

Dumbbell Calf Raise

PRIMARY TARGET MUSCLES: Calves

NOTES: This exercise is a good alternative for developing the calves if you don't have a calf-raise machine available. It can be done one leg at a time or both legs at once. The one-legged version uses one dumbbell at a time, while the two-legged version requires holding a dumbbell in each hand. Otherwise, execution is the same for both versions.

EXECUTION AND FORM

Step 1: Use a step or a couple of 25-pound barbell plates as a platform and position your feet a couple inches apart or one foot on each plate. The heels should hang off the platform. For the one-leg version, hold the non-working foot up behind you.

Step 2: Hold a dumbbell in each hand and let your arms hang at your side. For the one-leg version, hold a dumbbell in one hand and use the non-working hand to grab a stationary object and keep you balanced.

Step 3: Keep your knees pointing straight ahead and bent very slightly during the exercise. The bent-knee position can help stretch the calves in the lower position and will save your lower back in the upper position.

Step 4: Make sure to keep your body straight during the exercise. Be careful not to bend at the waist during any portion of the movement or hyperextend your back at the top of the movement. Doing either of these can injure your back. Stick your chest out and keep your shoulders squared at all times during the exercise. Keep your head straight and level, and look straight ahead at all times.

Step 5: Focus your attention on contracting your calf muscles. Really try to "feel" where the muscle is. Keeping your body as straight as possible, lower your heels toward the floor and slowly bring the calves to a full stretch. Hold this position for two seconds.

Step 6: From this position, without momentum, push off the balls of your feet and come up onto your tiptoes, pushing as high as possible. Concentrate on contracting the calves as hard as you can.

Step 7: Slowly lower your body to the stretch position, making sure the calf muscles endure the negative portion of the resistance. Do not allow your heels to drop too fast. Go slow and focus on the stretching of the calf muscles. If you're doing one leg at a time, do a full set with one leg then a set with the other leg. Always hold the dumbbell in the hand on the same side of your body as the calf that's being worked.

Dumbbell Calf Raise

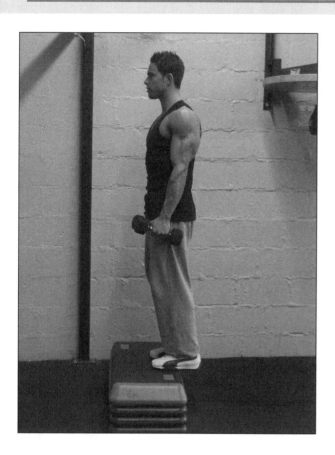

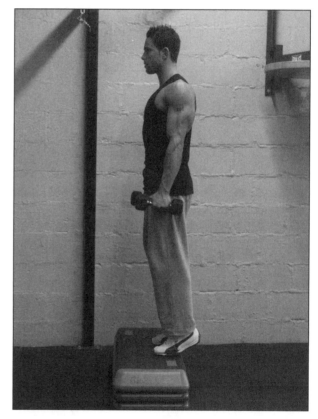

Mind Over Muscle Re-**MIND**-er:

Look upward and imagine that someone is dangling your favorite food overhead. The only way you can get it is by going as high on your toes as you can and grab a bite with your teeth. If you're against using food as a reward, it could be a hundred-dollar bill or something else as well—whatever motivates you to do the next rep.

Standing Calf Raise Machine

PRIMARY TARGET MUSCLES: Calves

> **NOTES:** The calf muscles are very stubborn and they won't respond to training unless you train them correctly. Besides needing different angles of training with proper technique and form, they also need a lot of weight and repetitions in order to grow. The standing calf raise machine is the easiest and safest way to load your calves up heavy. You can do this exercise one leg at a time or both legs at once. Execution for the exercise is the same for both versions.

EXECUTION AND FORM

Step 1: Set the weight to a resistance you can handle while practicing perfect form. Step on the platform and take hold of the grip bars on the sides of the shoulder harness. With your feet pointing straight ahead, place your toes and the balls of your feet on the edge of the platform with your heels hanging off. If using one leg at a time, hold the foot of your non-working leg up behind you.

Step 2: Set the shoulder pads so they will be slightly lower than your shoulders while you are in this position. Bend at the knees and position your shoulders underneath the shoulder pads comfortably. Stand up straight so that your shoulders lift the shoulder pads, which will in turn lift the weight plates up.

Step 3: Keep your knees pointing straight ahead and bent very slightly during the exercise. The bent-knee position can help stretch the calves in the lower position and will save your lower back in the upper position.

Step 4: Make sure to keep your body straight during the exercise. Be careful not to bend at the waist during any portion of the movement or hyperextend your back at the top of the movement. Doing either of these can injure your back. Stick your chest out and keep your shoulders squared at all times during the exercise. Keep your head straight and level and look straight ahead at all times.

Step 5: Focus your attention on contracting your calf muscles. Feel where the muscle is. Keeping your body as straight as possible, lower your heels toward the floor and slowly bring the calves to a full stretch. Hold this contraction.

Step 6: From this position, without momentum, contract the calves and push off the balls of your feet to come up onto your tiptoes. Push as high as possible and concentrate on contracting the calves as hard as you can.

Step 7: Slowly lower your body to the stretch position, making sure the calf muscles resist the weight on the way down. Do not allow your heels to drop too fast. Go slow and focus on the stretching of the calf muscles. If you're doing one leg at a time, do a full set with one leg then a set with the other leg.

Standing Calf Raise Machine

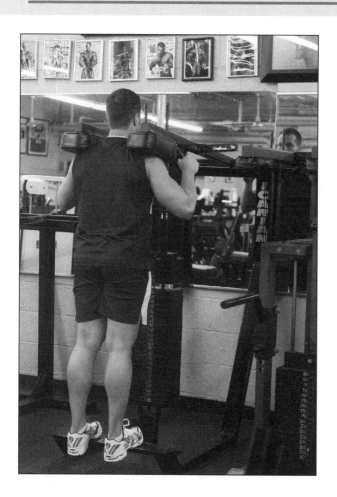

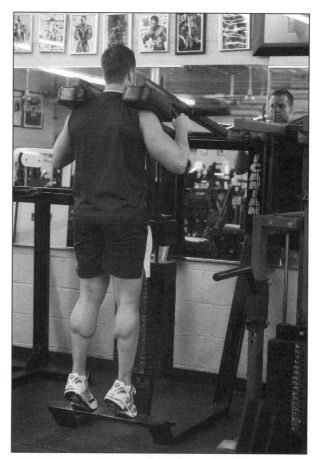

Mind Over Muscle Re-**MIND**-er:

Did you know that when contracting a muscle as hard as you can, the average person contracts only about 25 percent of the muscle fibers in that muscle? As you lift a weight, think about contracting the other 75 percent of those fibers. You won't recruit them all, but you'll definitely be able to recruit more than the norm. That will increase your strength during the exercise and, in turn, stimulate greater muscle growth.

Seated Calf Raise

PRIMARY TARGET MUSCLES: Lower Calf

NOTES: The seated position is especially great for those who have lower back pain. The soleus (lower calf) muscle becomes highly engaged, when the knee is bent. Do not allow your feet to bounce or gain momentum, as your heels dip towards the ground.

EXECUTION AND FORM

Step 1: Choose a weight with which you can practice perfect form. The object is to use good form rather than just trying to lift a gargantuan amount of weight. Sit down and position your feet on the platform with your feet pointing straight ahead, your toes and the balls of your feet on the platform, and your heels hanging off the platform.

Step 2: With your heels about halfway off the floor, place the padded support on top of your thighs. Make sure that it fits snug against the thigh, close to the knee rather than high on top of the thigh. Position your hands on the sides of the thigh pad.

Step 3: Keep your torso straight and do not lean forward or backward during the exercise. Keep your head straight and level, and look straight ahead at all times.

Step 4: Focus your attention on your calves. Flex them. Once you are in position and ready to begin the exercise, press your toes downward so that your knees raise up—and the weight with them. At the full height, release the catch and lower your heels toward the floor. Slowly bring the calves to a full stretch.

Step 5: From this position, without momentum, push off the balls of your feet and come up onto your

tiptoes, pushing as high as possible. Contract the calves as hard as you can and concentrate all of your efforts on the calves.

Step 6: Slowly begin lowering your heels back once again to the stretch position, making sure you make the calf muscles endure the negative portion of the resistance. Feel the contraction in your calves as they lower the weight and stretch out.

Step 7: As you reach the bottom position, with the heels pointing to the floor, make sure you do not allow your heels to drop too fast. Go slow and focus on the stretching of the calf muscles.

Seated Calf Raise

SECONDARY TARGET MUSCLES: **Upper Calf**

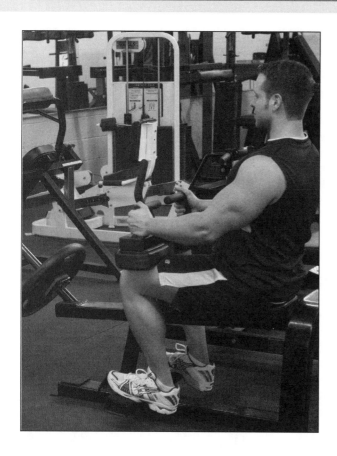

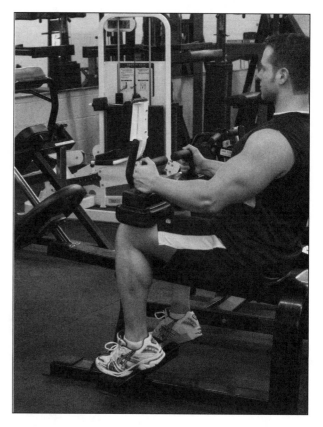

Mind Over Muscle Re-**MIND**-er:

During your pre-workout visualizations, don't forget to visualize the pain you're likely to feel in each exercise. Imagine the pain vividly. Then imagine how you are going to cope with it. With practice, this technique will make pain management automatic instead of "problematic."

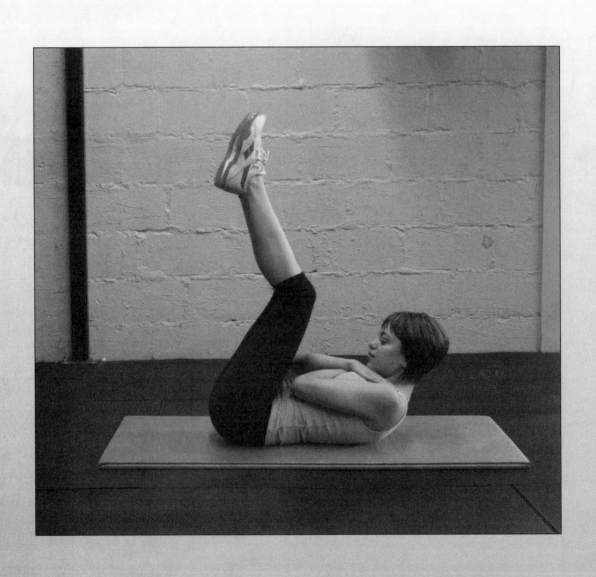

Abdominals

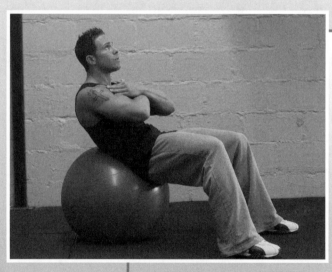

- Bicycle Crunch
- Knee-In
- Lying Leg Raise and Crunch
- Plank
- Swiss Ball Crunch
- V-Up

Bicycle Crunch

PRIMARY TARGET MUSCLES: **Obliques**

NOTES: Do not do this exercise with haste. Slow down to get the full range of motion and full contraction. A controlled pace also reduces risk of back injury. Do not use added resistance for this exercise.

EXECUTION AND FORM

Step 1: Lie on your back with your knees up and bent at 90 degrees, so that your thighs are perpendicular to the floor and your lower legs are parallel to it. Tuck your chin in and place your hands lightly behind your ears.

WARNING: Do not pull on your head during this exercise. It can cause neck injuries. If you find it difficult to avoid doing so, you can touch your fingertips to your deltoid muscles instead.

Step 2: Tighten up your abs with an isometric contraction and press your lower back to the floor.

Step 3: Simultaneously squeeze your right shoulder and left knee toward one another. Do not reach with your elbow as this can lessen the contraction of your abs. Your entire torso should twist and your right shoulder blade should come off the floor.

Step 4: Stop when you've crunched as far as you can, or when your elbow touches your knee.

Step 5: Now bring your left shoulder and right knee toward each other in the same way. Return to the starting position to complete one repetition. Again, twist the entire torso.

Step 6: Remember to keep your abs tight throughout the exercise. It's okay if your thighs extend a bit past perpendicular between crunches, but don't let your feet touch the floor. And always keep your lower back pressed to the floor to prevent injury.

Bicycle Crunch

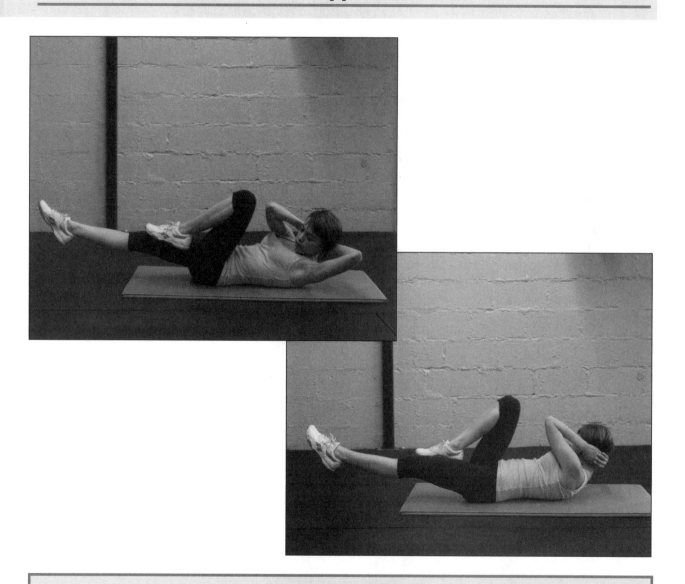

Mind Over Muscle Re-**MIND**-er:

Try counting your reps backward. Sometimes counting out the number of reps you have left makes it easier toward the end of the set because now your mind/muscle link is all about: "Only three more, I can handle it . . . only two more, I can do it . . . last one, this is easy!"

Knee-In

PRIMARY TARGET MUSCLES: **Lower Abdominals**

NOTES: Knee-ins are more convenient than some of the other lower abdominal exercises, but just as effective. This exercise gives you the ability to really squeeze the lower abs when the knees are brought in toward your chest. If the particular workout phase calls for a specific number of repetitions or added weight, you may either attach ankle weights to your ankles or place a weight plate between your feet. Just make sure to use a weight light enough to manage proper form and stay in control, but heavy enough to provide a challenge to the muscles.

EXECUTION AND FORM

Step 1: Sit on the floor or on the edge of a chair or exercise bench, with your legs extended in front of you. Your hands should be holding on to the sides of the bench or pressed to the floor for support.

Step 2: Keep your knees together and tense your abdominals and glutes. Contract your abs and pull the knees in toward your chest until you can go no farther. Hold the contraction.

Step 3: Keep tension on your lower abdominal muscles as you return to the start position. Repeat until you've reached your daily goal of sets.

Knee-In

SECONDARY TARGET MUSCLES: **Hip Adductors**

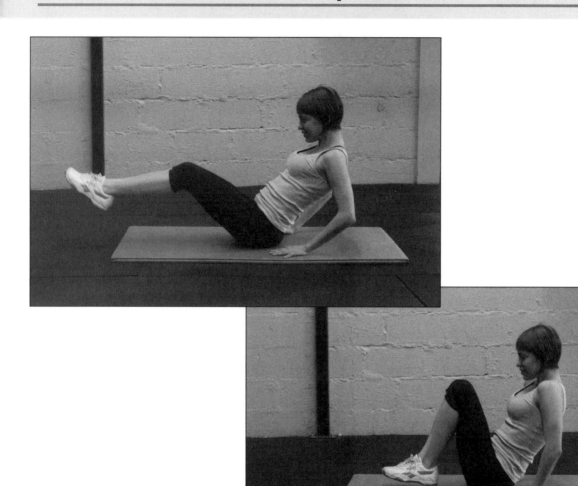

Mind Over Muscle Re-**MIND**-er:

Don't rush through this exercise. The goal for each rep is to slowly lower and raise your legs, which actually serve as the weight for this exercise, and feel every inch of your abdominals contracting. Don't let your hip flexors do the work here! By visualizing your abdominals contracting, you will resist the temptation to "shift your weight" to the hips.

Lying Leg Raise and Crunch

PRIMARY TARGET MUSCLES: Lower and Upper Abdominals

NOTES: Leg raises require more than simply lifting the legs off of the floor. Doing so can hurt the lower back and will do nothing to improve your lower abdominal muscles. You must focus and feel the abdominal muscles actually working while you raise your legs. Combining the leg raise with a crunch works the entire abdominal region at the same time. Do not use added resistance for this exercise.

EXECUTION AND FORM

Step 1: Lay flat on the floor with your legs straight out, except for a slight bend in the knees to help prevent lower back injury. Cross your hands over your chest.

Step 2: Tighten your abs and press your lower back to the floor. (This is a preventative measure against lower back injury.) If you find this difficult to do, contracting your glutes will help you.

Step 3: Begin by lifting your legs about five inches off the ground and holding. Meanwhile, tuck your chin into the collar bone. This is for preparation. Focus in on your abdominal muscles and isometrically contract them before you begin.

Step 4: Now you are going to do two things at the same time:
  a. Lift your legs straight up until they are perpendicular to the ground.
  b. Crunch your chest to your knees.

Your back and buttocks should both come slightly off the ground. Do not try to do this motion quickly; you will only overstress your lower back and possibly injure it. Remember to stay focused on your abdominal contraction and pressing your lower back to the ground.

Step 5: At full contraction, squeeze your abs as tight as you can.

Step 6: Slowly return the legs to the bottom position but remember to stop five inches from the floor. From here you will once again lift the legs. Do not let your lower back come up off the floor.

Lying Leg Raise and Crunch

SECONDARY TARGET MUSCLES: Hip Adductors

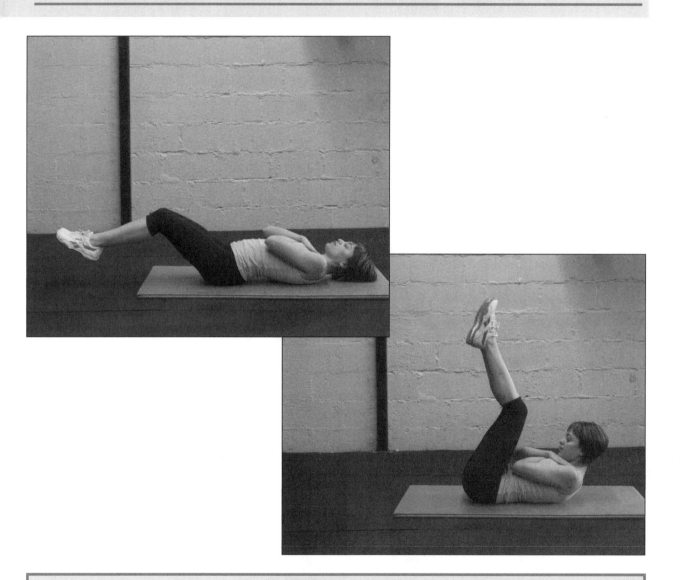

Mind Over Muscle Re-**MIND**-er:

Stay motivated during your workout by remembering your goals. Why, specifically, are you doing this? What will you be able to do once you have that six-pack of abs you're working so hard for? Picture it vividly in your mind and know that if you're going to have it, then you've got to work hard, hard, hard! (But you will surely get it soon!)

Plank

PRIMARY TARGET MUSCLES: Lower & Upper Abdominals

NOTES: Unlike other exercises in this section, the Plank is a static exercise, meaning you hold the contracted position for an extended period instead of doing repetitions. Therefore, the Two-Step Rep does not apply to this exercise. Although the Plank targets the entire abdominal region, it also does nearly as well to strengthen the lower back.

EXECUTION AND FORM

Step 1: Start on your hands and knees on the floor.

Step 2: Go down on your elbows, with your forearms lying on the floor, and clasp your hands together.

Step 3: To begin a set, raise your knees off the floor and straighten your body and legs. Your torso should form a straight line from your shoulders to your heels, and your bodyweight is supported on your elbows and toes.

Step 4: You can either look straight ahead or straight down during the exercise. In either case, keep your neck straight but relaxed. Hold the suspended position for a minute or more to complete the set.

Step 5: During the rest interval between sets lower your knees to the floor.

Plank

SECONDARY TARGET MUSCLES: **Erector Spinae (lower back)**

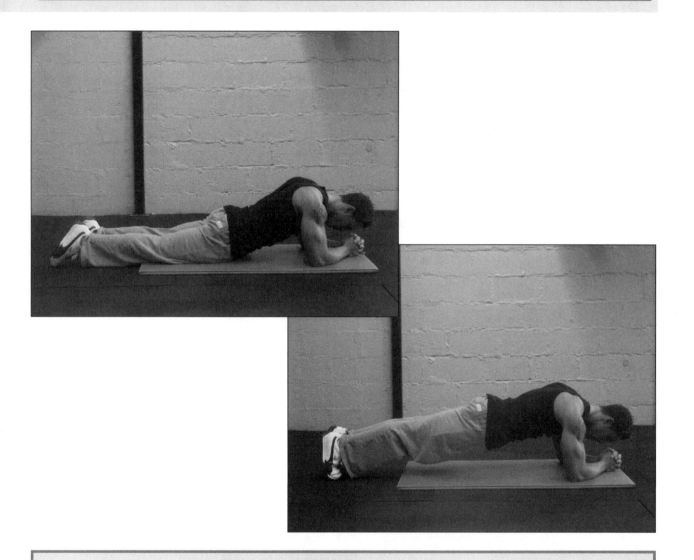

Mind Over Muscle Re-**MIND**-er:

The Full Body Tension Technique is a great device for this exercise, because your body becomes rigid and straight like an iron beam. Full Body Tension also reduces strain on the lower back because it receives assistance from surrounding muscle groups.

Swiss Ball Crunch

PRIMARY TARGET MUSCLES: Upper and Lower Abdominals

NOTES: Swiss Ball Crunches require more abdominal contraction than standard crunches on the floor, so you will probably not be able to do as many of these as you might be used to. If the particular workout phase calls for a specific number of repetitions or added weight, you may either place a weight plate on your chest or hold onto a pulley attachment during the movement. Just make sure to use a weight light enough to manage proper form and stay in control, but heavy enough to provide a challenge to the muscles.

EXECUTION AND FORM

Step 1: With your feet flat on the floor and knees at a 90-degree angle, lay back on a Swiss ball so that the ball supports your back and your butt is nearly hanging off the ball.

Step 2: With your hands crossed over your chest or placed behind the ears, stretch back over the Swiss ball.

Isometrically contract the abs before you begin the crunch and focus your concentration on that contraction.

Step 3: Without pulling on your head or neck, contract the abs and crunch your chest toward your pelvis. Exhale as you come up and raise your shoulder blades clear of the Swiss Ball.

Step 4: At the top position, contract the abs hard and hold. Return to the starting position using a controlled descent.

Swiss Ball Crunch

SECONDARY TARGET MUSCLES: Obliques

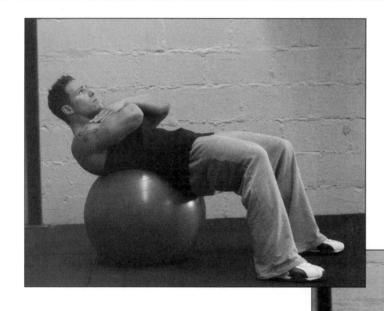

Mind Over Muscle Re-**MIND**-er:

The Full Body Tension technique can give more punch to your crunches. Your abs are the connecting link (core) of all of your body's musculature. By tensing the other muscles in your body, your abs have to resist their pull as well as the weight of your upper body, thereby providing maximum stimulus for the abdominals.

V-Up

PRIMARY TARGET MUSCLES: Lower & Upper Abdominals

NOTES: This is a very good incorporation exercise for the upper and lower abdominal muscles. You will notice that it is a variation of the crunch, but much more intense. You will simultaneously exercise the upper and lower abs. Do not use added resistance with this exercise.

EXECUTION AND FORM

Step 1: Sit on the floor, making sure you are lying on a carpet or mat. Put your arms by your side for support, slightly behind your torso.

Step 2: Raise your torso to a position 45 degrees off the floor. Keep the legs straight and flat on the ground. Focus on keeping the head and neck in line with your chest.

Step 3: Begin by isometrically contracting the abdominal muscles before moving.

Step 4: Crunch forward by moving your torso toward your feet (as if trying to make your chest touch your legs), while you lift your legs in a reverse crunch motion.

Step 5: The object is to simultaneously lift your legs and torso, thus crunching your mid-section. In the fully-contracted position, your legs should be raised about 12 inches off the floor. For maximum benefit, you must truly focus on the contraction of your abdominal muscles here. If you do, the contraction will be very intense.

Step 6: Slowly return to the start position, but do not allow your legs to touch the ground. This is a true measure of time under muscular tension and is very important if you want to obtain great results from your efforts.

Step 7: Without rest or momentum, slowly begin once again to lift your chest and legs to the fully contracted position.

V-Up

SECONDARY TARGET MUSCLES: **Hip Adductors**

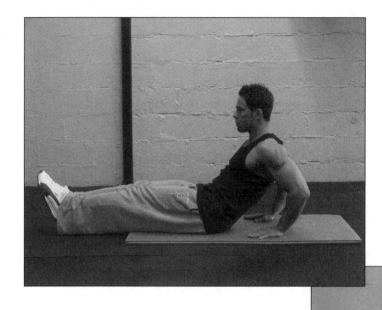

Mind Over Muscle Re-**MIND**-er:

Visualize your abdominals as a set of hydraulic pistons connecting your sternum to your thighs. On the contraction, the pistons pull the thighs and sternum toward each other just like the pistons on a back hoe or some other piece of construction equipment. Concentrate on the pull of those abdominal pistons.

PART THREE:

The Mind-Muscle Connection

Welcome to the part of the book where we present you with the routines that you will use to sculpt that physique and increase your *Mind Over Muscle* awareness and connection. By now you have been given a lot of tools, both philosophical and practical, with which to fine-tune the body of your dreams. But as I've said on numerous occasions, a vision without a plan is just a daydream. Here is where we arm you with a place, a time, and a plan so that you can go from dreaming about the body you've always wanted to achieving it.

The goal of these workouts is not only to get you in better shape, but also to teach you the correct way to fully feel the muscles working and the way to execute a proper routine for improving your mind-muscle connection. The routines include regimens for beginner, intermediate, and advanced levels of training. Please take note that the higher rep schemes are a way of challenging your body and stimulating growth, at any stage, and can be modified as such. For instance, to "shock" your system and jar your workouts doesn't require as many sets/reps as I might suggest for the advanced lifter, but you can certainly adapt them if you are a beginner or intermediate.

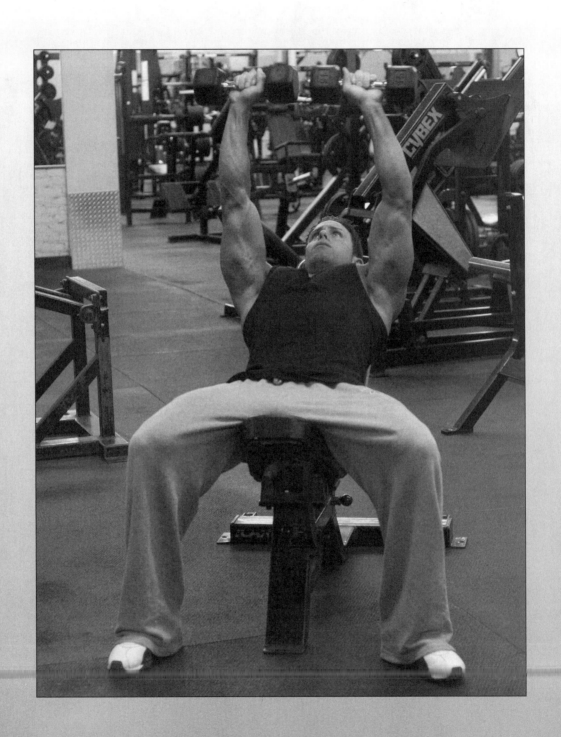

Chapter 9:

Your Plan of Action

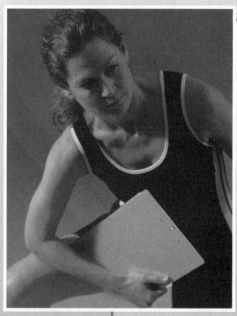

Now it's time to put all of the fantastic mindfulness exercises and muscle-building exercises into a unified plan of action. In order to make the most of your training, you will want to keep changing your workout routines so that you keep challenging your mind and body. This is called periodization.

How do you change your routine? There are many things you can do: add cardio at different times or intensities; change reps, sets, and weights; and keep in mind the three phases of training: Anatomical Adaptation, Hypertrophy, and Absolute Strength. In this section, I'll explain how to use each of these phases to reach your goals for your perfect body and mind.

No matter which kind of workout you are planning to do, don't forget to bring these three necessities for a great workout:

1. a towel
2. a watch
3. water

Cardio

As we have learned, cardiovascular training is essential for those of you who want to create a well-balanced body. Cardio training:

- Strengthens the heart
- Decreases depression and anxiety
- Decreases body fat, which helps to define muscles
- Prevents high blood pressure and lowers your resting heart rate
- Increases aerobic work capacity, allowing you to do more work with less strain on your heart
- Increases overall function, performance, and well-being.
- Enhances blood flow to working muscles, which in turn delivers more nutrients for optimal performance and growth.

The great thing about cardiovascular training is that you don't have to go overboard to realize the significant results. As with most people, you're probably also interested in losing excess body fat. If you are, the following information is ideal for getting into the fat-burn-zone. The recommended levels of performance are as follows:

Frequency: In general, cardio should be performed 3 to 5 times per week without more than 48 hours of rest passing between sessions. Any longer than 48 hours and your body starts to lose the positive effects of the previous session(s).

Duration: 20 to 60 minutes per session is sufficient for intermediate and advanced cardio fitness levels. For beginners, 1 to 2 small sessions of 10 to 12 minutes (not including warm up/cool down periods) should be performed for the first few weeks, then gradually increase the duration per

session each week thereafter as your body progresses.

Intensity: Using an appropriate intensity level is essential for obtaining significant results from any type of cardio activity. Beginners should work at a pace below 55 percent of their maximum heart rate for a few weeks to build a strong tolerance to the cardio activity before raising the intensity level. Intermediate and advanced individuals should work at a pace of 55 or 65 percent to 90 percent of their maximum heart rate.

So now you're wondering when is the best time to do your cardio training, right? My answer is "Anytime!" Whenever you have time available and feel your best, that's the best time to train—period! There is a lot of debate on whether you should train in the morning on an empty stomach. When you first wake up in the morning, your body is naturally lower in glycogen stores and void of carbohydrates. This state is said to be the optimum time for tapping into your triglycerides stores (fat energy) for energy. If this works for you, great!

I personally do my cardio training when I feel like it. That's right: if I wake up in the morning, am feeling good and have adequate energy, then the morning works for me. But I am typically not a morning person, so the ideal time for doing my cardio sessions is right after my weight training workout. I highly recommend that you do your cardio training after a weight training workout, rather than before.

Because the body relies on glucose for energy during a resistance training workout, by the time you are done with your weight training routine, your glucose reserves will be diminished and your body will be more than ready to tap into your triglyceride reserves (fat energy), during your cardio session.

However, if you are primarily interested in shedding body fat and staying fit, then I would say that doing your cardio before your weight training is fine. Just be aware that you will have less energy afterward and it could affect the intensity of your weight training sessions, which are always more effective when your energy is higher.

Yoga

Yoga is one of the earliest examples of human beings learning to tap into the mind-body connection. This powerful practice:

- Relaxes the mind and body
- Helps control your breath
- Increases flexibility and strength
- Improves your posture
- Boosts your energy level
- Strengthens your immune system

In addition, because yoga requires no equipment (although a yoga mat may be useful), you can do it anywhere and any time. I recommend that you start every day with a sun salutation to warm up and prepare your body and mind for the day to come. Also, add some yoga practices to your cardio sessions as part of your warm-up or cooldown periods.

Strength Training

Reps, Sets, and Weights
Choosing your reps, sets, and weights can be the most confusing part of strength training. How many reps and sets you do will depend on your individual goals. Here are a few general guidelines to help you determine what set and rep scheme will best meet your goals:

- **To lose body fat and build muscle:** Use enough weight that you can ONLY complete 10 to 12 repetitions per set. Do one to three sets (one for beginners, two to three for intermediate and advanced exercisers). Rest 30 to 60 seconds between sets and at least 2 days between workouts involving the same muscle groups.

- **For muscle gain:** Use enough weight that you can ONLY complete six to eight repetitions per set, and do three or more sets, resting for 1 to 2 minutes between sets and at least 2 days between sessions. For beginners, give yourself several weeks of conditioning before you tackle weight training with this degree of difficulty. You may need a spotter for many exercises.

- **For health and muscular endurance:** Use enough weight that you can ONLY complete 12 to 16 repetitions with good form in each set. Do one to three sets, resting 20 to 30 seconds between sets and at least 1 day between workout sessions.

- **To determine how much weight you should use:** Start with a light weight and perform one set. Continue adding weight until you can ONLY do the desired number of repetitions.

TRAINING WHILE TRAVELING

If you travel a lot, you'll want to be able to take your workout program with you so you can maintain it. Doing so is not difficult, but it does take some planning. Here are some options.

Find a fitness center: If you're staying a motel or hotel, find out if they have a fitness center. If not, ask someone if there is a nearby gym you can go to while you're there. If you find a gym or fitness center, you can pretty much stay with your regular exercises and just vary them depending on what machines are available. If the available machines don't allow you to do *exactly* the same exercises your routine calls for, don't use it as an excuse to not exercise at all and derail the good work you've done to date. Simply pick replacement exercises that target the same muscles or muscle groups. For example, you may not be able to do dumbbell rows, but you can probably do chins, cable rows, or upright rows and thus target the same muscle groups through this variety of accessible options.

Take equipment with you: This is most feasible if you are traveling by car. Bring along a pair of adjustable weight dumbbells and where your program calls for barbell or machine exercises, substitute dumbbell exercises that target the same muscles. For instance, instead of bench presses with a barbell, you might do floor presses (bench presses done on the floor rather than on a bench) with dumbbells. If you are using public transportation, such as a plane or a train, bringing dumbbells along is not a good option.

Resistance bands are a good substitute. There are several kinds of resistance bands available on the market. The best ones consist of two handles that allow you to connect lengths of rubber tubing between them. You can vary the resistance by changing the number of tubes that are used, or by using stronger or weaker tubing. Use the manual that comes with your resistance bands to determine which exercises to use in place of your normal workout exercises. Again, substitute exercises that target the same muscles.

Do bodyweight exercises: Bodyweight exercises don't allow you to isolate muscles the same way free weights and machines do. Because of that, you may have to do more sets and reps or more variations of an exercise to get the kind of workout that you're used to.

Whether you're using bodyweight exercises, machines at the hotel, or bringing your own equipment, the *Mind Over Muscle* principles, including Zone-Tone, visualization, and Two-Step Reps, still apply. For every exercise remember to focus, concentrate, and apply the Zone-Tone techniques before you begin each set. Remember, your weight set might not be fully portable, but your mind can take your body anywhere it wants to go.

Even to perfection!

WARNING: Do not try to add too much weight at this time! This is a time of identifying your limits and your abilities, of testing the waters, not diving in head first. I like to call it "a time of discovery." An advanced exerciser will have a great grasp on how much they can handle, however, they still need to be cautious of going overboard, where the weight is too great for their muscles to handle. You will hurt yourself by attempting to lift too much weight. By testing your initial limits you have set up a bench mark by which you will set and measure weight-lifting goals for the duration.

You've got your whole life to be a healthy, happy, fit individual; don't set yourself back a few weeks or months by getting jumpy right out of the gate. Allow yourself this time to ease into the transition. If your preliminary weight limit seems too low at first, just think of your initial limits as something that you will easily surpass once you get into the intermediate and advanced levels of your workout regimen.

Shock & Awe

Remember that your muscles grow while trying to adapt to a new work load. From time to time, your body needs a bit of "Shock & Awe" to keep it progressing properly. To avoid growing stale and hitting a plateau, try revising your routine every 12 weeks or so. Here's a list of 10 ways to change your routine to keep your muscles in shock:

1. Increase the weights you use by 10 percent.
2. Add another set of repetitions to each exercise.
3. Decrease your rest periods between sets.
4. Increase your rest periods between sets.
5. Increase the number of repetitions in each set.
6. Increase the weight of your exercises by 20 percent and do half as many reps in each set.
7. Change the tempo of your repetitions (See Two-Step Rep Technique).
8. Change the exercise for each muscle group, i.e. do barbell bench presses instead of dumbbell presses, or leg presses instead of squats.
9. Decrease the weight by 25 percent and do high-rep sets of 30 to 50.
10. Do single-repetition sets and increase the weight on each set until you can no longer do a rep with good form.

Three Phases of Training

As your body adapts to its training in process, it will undergo the three phases of training: Anatomical Adaptation, Hypertrophy, and Absolute Strength. This is called periodization. In the intermediate and advanced routines, I've given you the most efficient manipulation of sets, repetitions, and rest between sets in order to ensure maximum results. You will spend 1 week in the Anatomical Adaptation phase, 5 in the Hypertrophy phase, and 4 in the Absolute Strength phase, but as you'll see, the length of these phases can vary if you feel you need more time in a specific phase.

If you are a beginner, you need to spend more time in the Anatomical Adaptation phase to make sure that your body adapts thoroughly to the new stimuli of strength training. Therefore, the whole beginner routine in this book is a 6-week Anatomical Adaptation phase, after which you can go on to the intermediate routine and begin to let periodization work for you.

If you are new to working out, you would obviously begin with the beginner routine. If you are a weekend warrior, and have worked out here and there but not on a consistent or regular schedule, assess your current fitness level. If you are generally fit and feel comfortable with the exercises in the intermediate routine, then you may be able to start with the intermediate routine but just do an extra week or two of the Anatomical Adaptation phase. If you are not as fit or don't feel comfortable diving into the intermediate phase, start with the beginner phase first then move on to the intermediate phase. If you are a seasoned athlete but transitioning from another routine, gauge the

amount of time you need to recover from your last routine; again, you may decide you need to do an extra week or two of the Anatomical Adaptation phase.

PHASE 1:
Anatomical Adaptation

The main goal of this phase is to give the body a rest in order to allow it to catch up and recover from previous training. This weeklong phase is critical in order to prevent overtraining and overuse injuries. Typically, one week of this phase is good enough for the purposes described, though highly overtrained athletes or weekend warriors may require up to 2 and 3 weeks of this phase.

To assess whether or not you could use more

THE STOP-GO TECHNIQUE

Try this technique for high repetition training:

1. With an intention of reaching 25 reps, do as many reps as you can. If you reach muscular failure at, say, 12 repetitions, place the weight back on the rack, rest for 5 to 10 seconds and then do a few more reps with that same weight.

2. If your energy level is still adequate and you can handle the burn associated with lactic acid, you can do this a couple of more times without having to lessen the weight. If you do feel like you cannot do another few reps or the burn becomes just too much to handle with the same weight, take some weight off and keep going in the same manner, until you've reached the ultimate number of 25 repetitions.

or less time in the Anatomical Adaptation phase, listen to your body. Are you very tired? Achy? Weak? Have you lost motivation to train? All of these things could very well be a result of overtraining. If you are feeling any of these things, I recommend that you see your doctor to make sure these are not symptoms of a disease. If it turns out to just be overtraining, give yourself an extra week or two in this phase.

PHASE 2:
Hypertrophy
(Muscle Mass Increase)

The purpose of this phase is to increase muscle mass through high volume training performed with repetitions in the order, typically, of 10 to 12 (though one can go as low as 6 to 8). Rest periods in between sets are low in order to trigger maximum release of growth hormone and to prompt the body to store more energy substances in the muscle cell, such as creatine and glycogen. In the *Mind Over Muscle* intermediate and advanced routines, you'll spend 5 weeks in this phase. Five weeks is the minimum for this phase, since your body needs this much time to produce new muscle growth. If you want to add more muscle mass, you may extend this phase up to 8 weeks max. Don't go beyond 8 weeks! After that point, your body begins to adapt to the routine, and you risk overtraining and/or hitting a plateau.

PHASE 3:
Absolute Strength

Once muscle mass is increased, if one does not enter a phase where one teaches the body how to

maximally activate the new muscle fibers, one will reach a plateau and gains will cease to come. The goal of this phase is to increase your strength. Strength increases when, through the use of your nervous system, your body learns to activate more muscle fibers in order to move a specific load. This is accomplished by using heavier loads (or weight) at lower volume (or fewer reps). So you'll be doing just four to eight reps of each exercise but with heavier weights. This phase should last for 4 weeks—just enough time for your body to get used to the lower volume and heavier loads without overtraining or reaching a plateau.

Note that for Hypertrophy and Absolute Strength Phases for the intermediate and advanced routines, I like to include a full body routine at the end of the week with high repetitions in order to help expedite recovery. I like to call this the "Weekend Warrior" workout. The high repetitions force blood and nutrients into the muscle that will help recovery and create more capillaries that will deliver such items. Also, this trains the slow twitch oxidative fat-burning fibers in the body, which help to give you muscle endurance.

This is a higher volume, full-body workout. With this particular workout, you will do one to two sets per body part and anywhere from 15 to 25 repetitions per set. The 25-repetition set is great for bringing large amounts of blood and nutrients into your muscles. This "high intensity" protocol will help keep you motivated, help avoid the pitfalls associated with training plateaus, and is a great change of pace from the past week's workout. Incorporating both high and low repetition sets within your overall training routine allows you to work your muscles in different energy systems while still reaching your target repetition range and achieving your specific goals.

This high repetition workout is the perfect way to add an extra challenge to your routine. The worst thing a person can do is perform the same, redundant exercise protocol all the time. The human body has a profound ability to quickly adapt to a stimulus. If you exert the body through one type of training, without changing things up periodically, the body will quickly respond by adapting to that particular training and you will cease to see further results.

The trick is to challenge the muscles by altering the routine, the exercises, the weight load, the rep schemes, the set schemes, the speed of your reps, the rest time in between your sets, etc.

Chapter 10:

Beginner Routine

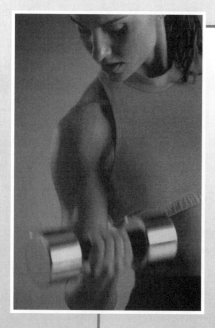

This routine is for those who have either no previous training experience or who are just coming back to the gym after a long period of inactivity. All you need to perform this routine is a pair of adjustable dumbbells and an adjustable bench with a leg extension/leg curl attachment. The goal of this routine is to gently introduce the body to the activity of weight training. This routine will allow the body to adapt to the stress without overtraining the body and shocking the system.

WEEKS 1-3

Special Instructions: Perform 3 days a week on non-consecutive days such as Monday/Wednesday/Friday or Tuesday/Thursday/Saturday. Alternate between Workouts 1 and 2; so one week you will do Workout 1 on Monday and Friday with Workout 2 performed on Wednesday. The following week, you will reverse this pattern.

WORKOUT 1	EXERCISE	Page No.	REPS	SETS	REST
	Incline Dumbbell Bench Press	70	12-15	2	1 min
	Flat Dumbbell Bench Press	66	12-15	2	1 min
	One-Arm Dumbbell Row	100	12-15	2	1 min
	Seated Machine Row (Palms facing forward)	104	12-15	2	1 min
	Bent-Over Lateral Raise	140	12-15	2	1 min
	Dumbbell Lateral Raise	138	12-15	2	1 min
	Dumbbell Concentration Curl	158	12-15	2	1 min
	Lying Dumbbell Triceps Extension	166	12-15	2	1 min

WORKOUT 2	EXERCISE	Page No.	REPS	SETS	REST
	Dumbbell Squat	186	12-15	2	1 min
	Leg Extension (Machine)	198	12-15	2	1 min
	Lying Leg Curl (Machine)	202	12-15	2	1 min
	Barbell or Dumbbell Lunge (Press with heels)	190, 192	12-15	2	1 min
	Dumbbell Calf Raise (One-Legged)	206	12-15	2	1 min
	Dumbbell Calf Raise (Two-Legged)	206	12-15	2	1 min
	Swiss Ball Crunch	222	15-25	2	1 min
	Knee-In	216	15-25	2	1 min

WEEKS 4-6

Special Instructions: Perform 3 days a week on non-consecutive days such as Monday/ Wednesday/Friday or Tuesday/Thursday/Saturday. Alternate between Workouts 1 and 2; so one week you will do Workout 1 on Monday and Friday with Workout 2 performed on Wednesday. The following week, you will reverse this pattern.

WORKOUT 1	EXERCISE	Page No.	REPS	SETS	REST
	Incline Dumbbell Bench Press	70	10-12	3	1 min
	Flat Dumbbell Bench Press	66	10-12	3	1 min
	One-Arm Dumbbell Row	100	10-12	3	1 min
	Seated Machine Row (Palms facing forward)	104	10-12	3	1 min
	Bent-Over Lateral Raise	140	10-12	3	1 min
	Dumbbell Lateral Raise	138	10-12	3	1 min
	Dumbbell Concentration Curl	158	10-12	3	1 min
	Lying Dumbbell Triceps Extension	166	10-12	3	1 min

WORKOUT 2	EXERCISE	Page No.	REPS	SETS	REST
	Dumbbell Squat	186	10-12	3	1 min
	Leg Extension (Machine)	198	10-12	3	1 min
	Lying Leg Curl (Machine)	202	10-12	3	1 min
	Barbell or Dumbbell Lunge (Press with heels)	190, 192	10-12	3	1 min
	Dumbbell Calf Raise (One-Legged)	206	10-12	3	1 min
	Dumbbell Calf Raise (Two-Legged)	206	10-12	3	1 min
	Swiss Ball Crunch	222	15-25	3	1 min
	Knee-In	216	15-25	3	1 min

Chapter 11:

Intermediate Routine

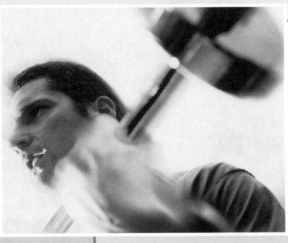

Home Gym Version

This routine is to be performed by those who have been training consistently for at least 6 months. All you need to perform this routine is a pair of adjustable dumbbells and an adjustable bench with a leg extension/leg curl attachment. For more variety and versatility, it would be best to also purchase an EZ Bar (Cambered bar) and/or a barbell, although you can use dumbbells for the barbell exercises if necessary.

WEEK 1: ANATOMICAL ADAPTATION

Special Instructions: Your goal this week is to give the body a rest so it can catch up and recover from previous training. Do this workout only 2 days a week, with several days in between (on Monday and Friday, for instance). Perform your reps in a rhythmic fashion, doing 1 rep per second without momentum.

WORKOUT 4	EXERCISE	Page No.	REPS	SETS	REST
FULL BODY	Incline Dumbbell Bench Press	70	15	2	2 min
	Flat Dumbbell Bench Press	66	15	2	2 min
	Two-Arm Dumbbell Row (Pronated Grip)	102	15	2	2 min
	Two-Arm Dumbbell Row (Neutral Grip)	102	15	2	2 min
	Dumbbell Shoulder Press	134	15	2	2 min
	Dumbbell Lateral Raise	138	15	2	2 min
	Bent-Over Lateral Raise	140	15	2	2 min
	Lying Leg Curl	202	15	2	2 min
	Leg Extension	198	15	2	2 min
	Dumbbell Calf Raise (Two-Legged)	206	15	2	2 min
	Bodyweight Squat	188	15	2	2 min
	Bicycle Crunch	214	15	2	2 min

WEEKS 2-6: HYPERTROPHY (MUSCLE MASS ACCUMULATION)

Special Instructions: Perform 4 days a week in the order specified. You can do Workouts 1 through 3 without taking any rest days in between, since they work different body parts, but I suggest that you take a day or two of rest before and after Workout 4. For instance, if you do Workouts 1 through 3 on Monday, Tuesday, and Wednesday, do Workout 4 on Friday. Use the Two-Step Rep tempo with all exercises.

WORKOUT 1	EXERCISE	Page No.	REPS	SETS	REST
CHEST ARMS	Incline Dumbbell Bench Press	70	10-12	3	1 min
	Flat Dumbbell Bench Press	66	10-12	3	1 min
	Incline Dumbbell Fly or Dumbbell Pullover	76	10-12	3	1 min
	Incline Dumbbell Curl	160	10-12	3	1 min
	Dumbbell Concentration Curl	158	10-12	3	1 min
	Overhead Dumbbell Extension	168	10-12	3	1 min
	Dumbbell Triceps Kickback	172	10-12	3	1 min

WORKOUT 2	EXERCISE	Page No.	REPS	SETS	REST
LEGS	Dumbbell Squat	186	10-12	3	1 min
	Leg Extension	198	10-12	3	1 min
	Barbell or Dumbbell Lunge	190, 192	10-12	3	1 min
	Lying Leg Curl	202	10-12	3	1 min
	Dumbbell Calf Raise (One-Legged)	206	10-12	3	1 min
	Dumbbell Calf Raise (Two-Legged)	206	10-12	3	1 min

WEEKS 2-6: HYPERTROPHY (MUSCLE MASS ACCUMULATION)

WORKOUT 3	EXERCISE	Page No.	REPS	SETS	REST
BACK **SHOULDERS** **ABS**	One-Arm Dumbbell Row	100	10-12	3	1 min
	Two-Arm Dumbbell Row (Pronated Grip)	102	10-12	3	1 min
	Two-Arm Dumbbell Row (Supinated Grip)	102	10-12	3	1 min
	Dumbbell Lateral Raise	138	10-12	3	1 min
	Bent-Over Lateral Raise	140	10-12	3	1 min
	E-Z Bar Upright Row	124	10-12	3	1 min
	Lying Leg Raise and Crunch	218	to failure	3	1 min

WORKOUT 4	EXERCISE	Page No.	REPS	SETS	REST
FULL **BODY**	Incline Dumbbell Bench Press	70	25	1	2 min
	Flat Dumbbell Bench Press	66	25	1	2 min
	Two-Arm Dumbbell Row (Pronated Grip)	102	25	1	2 min
	Two-Arm Dumbbell Row (Neutral Grip)	102	25	1	2 min
	Dumbbell Shoulder Press	134	25	1	2 min
	Dumbbell Lateral Raise	138	25	1	2 min
	Bent-Over Lateral Raise	140	25	1	2 min
	Lying Leg Curl	202	25	1	2 min
	Leg Extension	198	25	1	2 min
	Dumbbell Calf Raise (Two-Legged)	206	25	1	2 min
	Bodyweight Squat	188	25	1	2 min
	Bicycle Crunch	214	25*	1	2 min

* If you find 25 reps is too easy, add enough resistance so that you reach failure by 25 reps.

WEEKS 7-10: ABSOLUTE STRENGTH

Special Instructions: As with the Hypertrophy Phase, perform 4 days a week in the order specified. You can do Workouts 1 through 3 without taking any rest days in between, since they work different body parts, but I suggest that you take a day or two of rest before and after Workout 4. For instance, if you do Workouts 1 through 3 on Monday, Tuesday, and Wednesday, do Workout 4 on Friday. Use the Two-Step Rep tempo with all exercises.

WORKOUT 1	EXERCISE	Page No.	REPS	SETS	REST
CHEST **ARMS**	Incline Dumbbell Bench Press	70	8,6,5,4	4	1 min
	Flat Dumbbell Bench Press	66	8,6,5,4	4	1 min
	Incline Dumbbell Fly or Dumbbell Pullover	84, 76	8,6,5,4	4	1 min
	Incline Dumbbell Curl	160	8,6,5,4	4	1 min
	Dumbbell Concentration Curl	158	8,6,5,4	4	1 min
	Overhead Dumbbell Extension	168	8,6,5,4	4	1 min
	Dumbbell Triceps Kickback	172	8,6,5,4	4	1 min

WORKOUT 2	EXERCISE	Page No.	REPS	SETS	REST
LEGS	Dumbbell Squat	186	8,6,5,4	4	1 min
	Leg Extension	198	8,6,5,4	4	1 min
	Barbell or Dumbbell Lunge	190, 192	8,6,5,4	4	1 min
	Lying Leg Curl	202	8,6,5,4	4	1 min
	Dumbbell Calf Raise (One-Legged)	206	8,6,5,4	4	1 min
	Dumbbell Calf Raise (Two-Legged)	206	8,6,5,4	4	1 min

WEEKS 7-10: ABSOLUTE STRENGTH

You'll see that the workouts are similar to those in the Hypertrophy Phase except you'll add weight and reduce the reps with each set. Perform 4 sets of 8, 6, 5, 4 repetitions, unless otherwise specified, using the "Two-Step-Rep" repetition tempo. In other words, the first set you perform 8 reps, then you rest 1 minute, add weight and perform 6 reps. Rest 1 minute, add more weight and do 5 reps. Finally, rest 1 minute, add more weight, and do 4 reps.

WORKOUT 3	EXERCISE	Page No.	REPS	SETS	REST
BACK **SHOULDERS** **ABS**	One-Arm Dumbbell Row	100	8,6,5,4	3	1 min
	Two-Arm Dumbbell Row (Pronated Grip)	102	8,6,5,4	3	1 min
	Two-Arm Dumbbell Row (Supinated Grip)	102	8,6,5,4	3	1 min
	Dumbbell Lateral Raise	138	8,6,5,4	3	1 min
	Bent-Over Lateral Raise	140	8,6,5,4	3	1 min
	E-Z Bar Upright Row	124	8,6,5,4	3	1 min
	Lying Leg Raise and Crunch	218	8,6,5,4	3	1 min

WORKOUT 4	EXERCISE	Page No.	REPS	SETS	REST
FULL **BODY**	Incline Dumbbell Bench Press	70	25	1	2 min
	Flat Dumbbell Bench Press	66	25	1	2 min
	Two-Arm Dumbbell Row (Pronated Grip)	102	25	1	2 min
	Two-Arm Dumbbell Row (Neutral Grip)	102	25	1	2 min
	Dumbbell Shoulder Press	134	25	1	2 min
	Dumbbell Lateral Raise	138	25	1	2 min
	Bent-Over Lateral Raise	140	25	1	2 min
	Lying Leg Curl	202	25	1	2 min
	Leg Extension	198	25	1	2 min
	Dumbbell Calf Raise (Two-Legged)	206	25	1	2 min
	Bodyweight Squat	188	25	1	2 min
	Bicycle Crunch	214	25*	1	2 min

* If you find 25 reps is too easy, add enough resistance so that you reach failure by 25 reps.

WEEK 1: ANATOMICAL ADAPTATION

Commercial Gym Version

This routine is to be performed at a commercial gym by those who have been training consistently for at least 6 months.

Special Instructions: Your goal this week is to give the body a rest so it can catch up and recover from previous training. Do this workout only 2 days a week, with several days in between (on Monday and Friday, for instance). Perform your reps in a rhythmic fashion, doing 1 rep per second without momentum.

WORKOUT 4	EXERCISE	Page No.	REPS	SETS	REST
FULL BODY	Incline Dumbbell Bench Press	70	15	1	2 min
	Flat Dumbbell Bench Press	66	15	1	2 min
	Two-Arm Dumbbell Row (Pronated Grip)	102	15	1	2 min
	Two-Arm Dumbbell Row (Neutral Grip)	102	15	1	2 min
	Dumbbell Shoulder Press	134	15	1	2 min
	Dumbbell Lateral Raise	138	15	1	2 min
	Bent-Over Lateral Raise	140	15	1	2 min
	Lying Leg Curl	202	15	1	2 min
	Leg Extension	198	15	1	2 min
	Dumbbell Calf Raise (Two-Legged)	206	15	1	2 min
	Bodyweight Squat	188	15	1	2 min
	Bicycle Crunch	214	15*	1	2 min

* If you find 15 reps is too easy, add enough resistance so that you reach failure by 15 reps.

WEEKS 2-6: HYPERTROPHY (MUSCLE MASS ACCUMULATION)

Special Instructions: Perform 4 days a week in the order specified. You can do Workouts 1 through 3 without taking any rest days in between, since they work different body parts, but I suggest that you take a day or two of rest before and after Workout 4. For instance, if you do Workouts 1 through 3 on Monday, Tuesday, and Wednesday, do Workout 4 on Friday. Use the Two-Step Rep tempo with all exercises.

WORKOUT 1 CHEST ARMS	EXERCISE	Page No.	REPS	SETS	REST
	Incline Dumbbell Bench Press	70	10-12	3	1 min
	Flat Dumbbell Bench Press	66	10-12	3	1 min
	Incline Dumbbell Fly or Dumbbell Pullover	84, 76	10-12	3	1 min
	Incline Dumbbell Curl	160	10-12	3	1 min
	Dumbbell Concentration Curl	158	10-12	3	1 min
	Overhead Dumbbell Extension	168	10-12	3	1 min
	Pulley Triceps Kickback	174	10-12	3	1 min

WORKOUT 2 LEGS	EXERCISE	Page No.	REPS	SETS	REST
	Barbell Squat	184	10-12	3	1 min
	Barbell Squat (Wide Stance)	184	10-12	3	1 min
	Leg Extension	198	10-12	3	1 min
	Barbell or Dumbbell Lunge	190, 192	10-12	3	1 min
	Lying Leg Curl	202	10-12	3	1 min
	Standing Calf Raise Machine	208	10-12	3	1 min
	Seated Calf Raise	210	10-12	3	1 min

WEEKS 2-6: HYPERTROPHY (MUSCLE MASS ACCUMULATION)

WORKOUT 3 BACK SHOULDERS ABS	EXERCISE	Page No.	REPS	SETS	REST
	Wide Grip Pullup	112	10-12	3	1 min
	Close Reverse Grip Pulldown	120	10-12	3	1 min
	Low Pulley Row	108	10-12	3	1 min
	Dumbbell Lateral Raise	138	10-12	3	1 min
	Rear Deltoid Machine	142	10-12	3	1 min
	Dumbbell Upright Row	126	10-12	3	1 min
	Lying Leg Raise and Crunch	218	to failure	3	1 min

WORKOUT 4 FULL BODY	EXERCISE	Page No.	REPS	SETS	REST
	Incline Dumbbell Bench Press	70	25	1	2 min
	Flat Dumbbell Bench Press	66	25	1	2 min
	Wide Grip Pulldown	116	25	1	2 min
	Low Pulley Row (Neutral Grip)	108	25	1	2 min
	Dumbbell Shoulder Press	134	25	1	2 min
	Dumbbell Lateral Raise	138	25	1	2 min
	Rear Deltoid Machine	142	25	1	2 min
	Lying Leg Curl	202	25	1	2 min
	Leg Extension	198	25	1	2 min
	Calf Press	204	25	1	2 min
	Bodyweight Squat	188	25	1	2 min
	Bicycle Crunch	214	25*	1	2 min

* If you find 25 reps is too easy, add enough resistance so that you reach failure by 25 reps.

WEEKS 7-10: ABSOLUTE STRENGTH

Special Instructions: As with the Hypertrophy Phase, perform 4 days a week in the order specified. You can do Workouts 1 through 3 without taking any rest days in between, since they work different body parts, but I suggest that you take a day or two of rest before and after Workout 4. For instance, if you do Workouts 1 through 3 on Monday, Tuesday, and Wednesday, do Workout 4 on Friday. Use the Two-Step Rep tempo with all exercises.

WORKOUT 1	EXERCISE	Page No.	REPS	SETS	REST
CHEST ARMS	Incline Dumbbell Bench Press	70	8,6,5,4	4	1 min
	Flat Dumbbell Bench Press	66	8,6,5,4	4	1 min
	Incline Dumbbell Fly or Dumbbell Pullover	76	8,6,5,4	4	1 min
	Preacher Curl	156	8,6,5,4	4	1 min
	Reverse E-Z Curl	152	8,6,5,4	4	1 min
	Close Grip Bench Press	164	8,6,5,4	4	1 min
	Triceps Pushdown	176	8,6,5,4	4	1 min

WORKOUT 2	EXERCISE	Page No.	REPS	SETS	REST
LEGS	Barbell Squat	184	8,6,5,4	4	1 min
	Barbell Squat (Wide Stance)	184	8,6,5,4	4	1 min
	Leg Extension	198	8,6,5,4	4	1 min
	Wide Stance Leg Press	196	8,6,5,4	4	1 min
	Standing Leg Curl	200	8,6,5,4	4	1 min
	Calf Press	204	8,6,5,4	4	1 min
	Standing Calf Raise Machine	208	8,6,5,4	4	1 min

WEEKS 7-10: ABSOLUTE STRENGTH

WORKOUT 3	EXERCISE	Page No.	REPS	SETS	REST
BACK **SHOULDERS** **ABS**	Wide Grip Pullup	112	8,6,5,4	4	1 min
	T-Bar Row	94	8,6,5,4	4	1 min
	High Pulley V-Bar Pulldown	118	8,6,5,4	4	1 min
	Dumbbell Lateral Raise	138	8,6,5,4	4	1 min
	Bent-Over Lateral Raise	140	8,6,5,4	4	1 min
	Barbell Shoulder Press	132	8,6,5,4	4	1 min
	Lying Leg Raise and Crunch	218	to failure	3	1 min

WORKOUT 4	EXERCISE	Page No.	REPS	SETS	REST
FULL **BODY**	Incline Dumbbell Bench Press	70	25	1	2 min
	Flat Dumbbell Bench Press	66	25	1	2 min
	Close Reverse Grip Pulldown	120	25	1	2 min
	T-Bar Row	94	25	1	2 min
	Dumbbell Shoulder Press	134	25	1	2 min
	Dumbbell Lateral Raise	138	25	1	2 min
	Bent-Over Lateral Raise	140	25	1	2 min
	Lying Leg Curl	202	25	1	2 min
	Leg Extension	198	25	1	2 min
	Seated Calf Raise	210	25	1	2 min
	Leg Press	104	25	1	2 min
	Bicycle Crunch	214	25*	1	2 min

* If you find 25 reps is too easy, add enough resistance so that you reach failure by 25 reps.

Chapter 12:

Advanced Routine

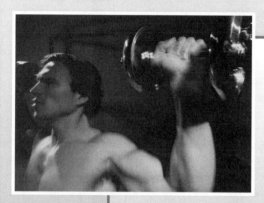

This routine is to be performed at a commercial gym by those who have been training consistently for at least a year. In order to engage and train each muscle to full development, it is necessary to do a variety of exercises using different positions, angles, and machines, so at this stage in your training you really need to have every piece of training apparatus at your beck and call. It would be virtually impossible to get all of that at home, unless your last name is Gold or Gates.

WEEK 1: ANATOMICAL ADAPTATION

Special Instructions: Your goal this week is to give the body a rest so it can catch up and recover from previous training. Do this workout only 2 days a week, with several days in between (on Monday and Friday, for instance). Perform your reps in a rhythmic fashion, doing 1 rep per second without momentum.

WORKOUT 4	EXERCISE	Page No.	REPS	SETS	REST
FULL BODY	Incline Barbell Bench Press	68	15	1	2 min
	Flat Barbell Bench Press	64	15	1	2 min
	Wide Grip Pullup	112	15	1	2 min
	Standing High Pulley V-Bar Row	110	15	1	2 min
	Barbell Shoulder Press	132	15	1	2 min
	Dumbbell Lateral Raise	138	15	1	2 min
	Rear Deltoid Machine	142	15	1	2 min
	Lying Leg Curl	202	15	1	2 min
	Leg Extension	198	15	1	2 min
	Calf Press	204	15	1	2 min
	Leg Press	194	15	1	2 min
	Bicycle Crunch	214	15	1	2 min

WEEKS 2-6: HYPERTROPHY (MUSCLE MASS ACCUMULATION)

Special Instructions: Perform 6 days a week in the order specified. You can do Workouts 1 through 5 without taking any rest days in between, since they work different body parts, but I suggest that you take a day of rest before or after Workout 6. For instance, work out Monday through Saturday, then rest on Sunday. Use the Two-Step Rep tempo with all exercises.

WORKOUT 1 BACK	EXERCISE	Page No.	REPS	SETS	REST
	Wide Grip Pullup (Overhand Grip)	112	10-12	4	1 min
	One-Arm Dumbbell Row or Plate-Loaded One-Arm Row (Neutral Grip)	100, 106	10-12	4	1 min
	Barbell Row (Pronated Grip) or T-Bar Machine Row	92, 96	10-12	4	1 min
	Standing High Pulley V-Bar Row or Narrow Grip V-Bar Pullup	110, 114	10-12	4	1 min
	Deadlift	88	10-12	4	1 min
	Swiss Ball Crunch	222	to failure	4	1 min
	Knee-In	216	to failure	4	1 min

WORKOUT 2 CHEST	EXERCISE	Page No.	REPS	SETS	REST
	Incline Barbell Bench Press	68	10-12	4	1 min
	Flat Barbell Bench Press or Flat Dumbbell Bench Press	64, 66	10-12	4	1 min
	Incline Dumbbell Bench Press (Palms facing)	70	10-12	4	1 min
	Chest Dip or Dumbbell Pullover	78, 76	10-12	4	1 min
	Flat Dumbbell Fly	82	10-12	4	1 min
	Flat Barbell Bench Press (Wide Grip)	64	10-12	4	1 min

WEEKS 2-6: HYPERTROPHY (MUSCLE MASS ACCUMULATION)

WORKOUT 3 LEGS	EXERCISE	Page No.	REPS	SETS	REST
	Barbell Lunge	190	10-12	4	1 min
	Barbell Squat	184	10-12	4	1 min
	Leg Extension	198	10-12	4	1 min
	Lying Leg Curl or Standing Leg Curl (One-Legged)	202, 200	10-12	4	1 min
	Seated Calf Raise or Calf Press	210, 204	10-12	4	1 min
	Bicycle Crunch	214	to failure	4	1 min

WORKOUT 4 SHOULDERS TRAPS	EXERCISE	Page No.	REPS	SETS	REST
	Barbell Shoulder Press	132	10-12	4	1 min
	Dumbbell Shoulder Press	134	10-12	4	1 min
	Dumbbell Lateral Raise	138	10-12	4	1 min
	Rear Deltoid Machine	142	10-12	4	1 min
	E-Z Bar Upright Row	124	10-12	4	1 min
	Dumbbell Shrug	128	10-12	4	1 min
	Smith Machine Shrug	130	10-12	4	1 min

WEEKS 2-6: HYPERTROPHY (MUSCLE MASS ACCUMULATION)

WORKOUT 5 ARMS	EXERCISE	Page No.	REPS	SETS	REST
	Overhead Rope Triceps Extension	170	10-12	4	1 min
	Barbell Curl	148	10-12	4	1 min
	Overhead Dumbbell Extension or Machine Triceps Extension	168, 178	10-12	4	1 min
	Dumbbell Triceps Kickback or Pulley Triceps Kickback	172, 174	10-12	4	1 min
	High Pulley Biceps Curl (One-Arm or Two-Arm)	162	10-12	4	1 min
	Lying Leg Raise and Crunch	218	to failure	4	1 min

WORKOUT 6 FULL BODY	EXERCISE	Page No.	REPS	SETS	REST
	Incline Barbell Bench Press	68	25	1	2 min
	Flat Barbell Bench Press	64	25	1	2 min
	Wide Grip Pullup	112	25	1	2 min
	Standing High Pulley V-Bar Row	110	25	1	2 min
	Barbell Shoulder Press	132	25	1	2 min
	Dumbbell Lateral Raise	138	25	1	2 min
	Rear Deltoid Machine	142	25	1	2 min
	Lying Leg Curl	202	25	1	2 min
	Leg Extension	198	25	1	2 min
	Standing Calf Raise Machine	208	25	1	2 min
	Lying Leg Curl	202	25	1	2 min
	Bicycle Crunch	214	25*	1	2 min

WEEKS 7-10: ABSOLUTE STRENGTH

Special Instructions: As with the Hypertrophy Phase, perform 6 days a week in the order specified. You can do Workouts 1 through 5 without taking any rest days in between, since they work different body parts, but I suggest that you take a day of rest before or after Workout 6. For instance, work out Monday through Saturday, then rest on Sunday. Use the Two-Step Rep tempo with all exercises.

WORKOUT 1 BACK	EXERCISE	Page No.	REPS	SETS	REST
	Wide Grip Pullup	112	8,6,5,4	4	1 min
	One-Arm Dumbbell Row or Plate-Loaded One-Arm Row (Neutral Grip)	100, 106	8,6,5,4	4	1 min
	Barbell Row (Pronated Grip) or T-Bar Machine Row	92, 96	8,6,5,4	4	1 min
	Standing High Pulley V-Bar Row or Narrow Grip V-Bar Pullup	110, 114	8,6,5,4	4	1 min
	Deadlift	88	8,6,5,4	4	1 min
	Swiss Ball Crunch	222	to failure	4	1 min
	Knee-In	216	to failure	4	1 min

WORKOUT 2 CHEST	EXERCISE	Page No.	REPS	SETS	REST
	Incline Barbell Bench Press	68	8,6,5,4	4	1 min
	Flat Barbell Bench Press or Flat Dumbbell Bench Press	64, 66	8,6,5,4	4	1 min
	Incline Dumbbell Bench Press (Palms facing)	70	8,6,5,4	4	1 min
	Chest Dip or Dumbbell Pullover	78, 76	8,6,5,4	4	1 min
	Flat Dumbbell Fly	82	8,6,5,4	4	1 min
	Flat Barbell Bench Press (Wide Grip)	64	8,6,5,4	4	1 min

WEEKS 7-10: ABSOLUTE STRENGTH

You'll see that the workouts are similar to those in the Hypertrophy Phase except you'll add weight and reduce the reps with each set. Perform 4 sets of 8, 6, 5, 4 repetitions, unless otherwise specified, using the "Two-Step-Rep" repetition tempo. In other words, the first set you perform 8 reps, then you rest 1 minute, add weight and perform 6 reps. Rest 1 minute, add more weight and do 5 reps. Finally, rest 1 minute, add more weight, and do 4 reps.

WORKOUT 3 LEGS	EXERCISE	Page No.	REPS	SETS	REST
	Barbell Lunge	190	8,6,5,4	4	1 min
	Barbell Squat	184	8,6,5,4	4	1 min
	Leg Extension	198	8,6,5,4	4	1 min
	Lying Leg Curl or Standing Leg Curl (One-Legged)	202, 200	8,6,5,4	4	1 min
	Barbell Squat (Wide Stance)	184	8,6,5,4	4	1 min
	Seated Calf Raise or Calf Press	210, 204	8,6,5,4	4	1 min
	Bicycle Crunch	214	8,6,5,4	4	1 min

WORKOUT 4 SHOULDERS TRAPS	EXERCISE	Page No.	REPS	SETS	REST
	Barbell Shoulder Press	132	8,6,5,4	4	1 min
	Dumbbell Shoulder Press	134	8,6,5,4	4	1 min
	Dumbbell Lateral Raise	138	8,6,5,4	4	1 min
	Rear Deltoid Machine	142	8,6,5,4	4	1 min
	Dumbbell Upright Row	126	8,6,5,4	4	1 min
	Dumbbell Shrug	128	8,6,5,4	4	1 min
	Smith Machine Shrug	130	8,6,5,4	4	1 min

WEEKS 7-10: ABSOLUTE STRENGTH

WORKOUT 5	EXERCISE	Page No.	REPS	SETS	REST
ARMS	Overhead Rope Triceps Extension	170	8,6,5,4	4	1 min
	Barbell Curl	148	8,6,5,4	4	1 min
	Overhead Dumbbell Extension or Machine Triceps Extension	168, 178	8,6,5,4	4	1 min
	Incline Dumbbell Curl or Hammer Curl	160, 154	8,6,5,4	4	1 min
	Dumbbell Triceps Kickback or Pulley Triceps Kickback	172, 174	8,6,5,4	4	1 min
	High Pulley Biceps Curl (One-Arm or Two-Arm)	162	8,6,5,4	4	1 min
	Lying Leg Raise and Crunch	218	to failure	4	1 min

WORKOUT 6	EXERCISE	Page No.	REPS	SETS	REST
FULL BODY	Incline Barbell Bench Press	68	25	1	2 min
	Flat Barbell Bench Press	64	25	1	2 min
	Wide Grip Pullup	112	25	1	2 min
	Standing High Pulley V-Bar Row	110	25	1	2 min
	Barbell Shoulder Press	132	25	1	2 min
	Dumbbell Lateral Raise	138	25	1	2 min
	Rear Deltoid Machine	142	25	1	2 min
	Lying Leg Curl	202	25	1	2 min
	Leg Extension	198	25	1	2 min
	Standing Calf Raise Machine	208	25	1	2 min
	Leg Press	194	25	1	2 min
	Bicycle Crunch	214	25	1	2 min

Conclusion

Mindful Results

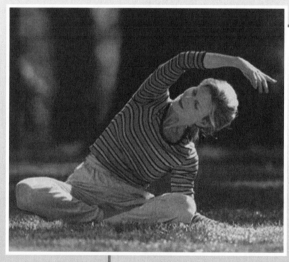

Pay Day—Get Ready For Results

Can you believe it? Our time together is finally at an end. It's been a long and winding road, and I'm sure there was a twist or a turn back there you didn't expect, but all in all I trust you've learned plenty and exercised more, and for that I think we are both thankful!

At times I know you wanted to close your mind to new realities and go back to your old comfort zone. Occasionally I know you were frustrated and had to read some sections twice, while wanting to skip others altogether. I even recognize that some of the information I've presented here was hard for you to swallow, considering the way it bucked the traditional paradigm of most exercise and nutrition books on the market today.

I respect and admire you for making it through to the end with me. I applaud your decision to stick with it and get here, but in fact it's you who should be impressed. No matter which of the *Mind Over Muscle* principles stays with you, no matter what "sticks," I want you to remember that just taking the first all-important step and reading this book, cover to cover, means that you are now one step closer to achieving your ultimate fitness goals.

If you follow every aspect of the program you will find that not only can you perform better with physical fitness, but you will also see other elements of your life change for the positive as well. Your confidence level increases even as your willpower elevates. You will sleep better, wake up refreshed, and start the day more positively than ever before. Negativity is a thing of the past and hopefully your newfound positive attitude will rub off on other people who are in the same situation you were in before this program.

Along these lines, please feel free to share this information with those whose lives you touch on a daily basis. In other words, this is not privileged information. First and foremost, I want you to benefit from the program. But much like this philosophy has been melded from my years of both teaching and learning, I was motivated to share it with others because it's worked so well for me. I would be honored to pass that torch along to you!

We have come a long way and I know we both have farther to go. One thing I've tried to stress throughout this book is that there is no end to the journey, but in fact the "journey is all." We establish one goal, reach it, establish a new goal, and move on. The goal is never "the end," but only the beginning of a new and more valuable goal.

There is no schedule but the one you create for yourself. There are no rules but the ones that you know will provide for the best results—*when you are ready.* You have the power over your success or your failure. I look forward to hearing how you do, and will look for you at book signings, seminars, classes, at the gym, and on my website.

Good luck and, as I tell my clients, "Believe and Achieve!"

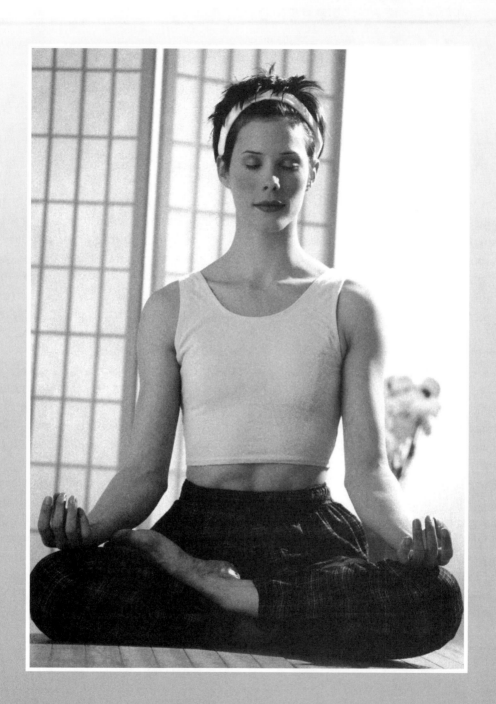

APPENDIX A:
My *Mind Over Muscle* Journal:

Thoughts for Creating Your Greatest Body Ever—

in the Shortest Amount of Time

I've included here a complimentary *Mind Over Muscle* Journal just for you. Don't worry: nobody will read it, grade it, judge it, approve of it or, for that matter, disapprove of it. I want you to feel free to write exactly what you feel, safe in the knowledge that your thoughts, your feelings, your emotions are "for your eyes only" and not for public scrutiny.

It's not difficult, but it's quite constructive. I keep a journal like this for myself and have found it quite useful over the past few years. In fact, it's quite simple: each day begins with a problem and ends with a solution. You pick the problems, and come back to the solutions.

For example, a problem of the day might be something to the effect of "I couldn't focus today, I wasn't 'fully there' and I should have been!" That's a common problem, but one with a myriad of solutions. In fact, your solution might be something as simple as, "I started the process of exercis-

ing without using my earphones. From this day forward I'm going to listen to my body instead!"

After each solution, I've provided space for you to write any general thoughts, plans, emotions, or concerns you have in the wake of this development. Personally, I use this space to set myself up for the next day's problem, but it's a "free space" and you should feel comfortable using it in any way you see fit.

I've included just one blank page here that you can photocopy as many times as you need. I suggest that you try to keep the journal for at least 30 days. It takes about a month for most people to experience real, lasting change in their bodies and their minds. This way, you've got the time to absorb what you read here and apply it to your daily life. But any amount of time you spend with it can help—and you might even find that you like it so much, you want to keep writing in your journal beyond your 30 days.

Date:

Time:

Problem of the Day: _____

_____

_____

_____

_____

_____

_____

_____

_____

_____

Solution of the Day: _____

_____

_____

_____

_____

_____

_____

_____

_____

_____

_____

General Thoughts: _____

_____

_____

_____

_____

_____

_____

_____

_____

APPENDIX B:
My *Mind Over Muscle* Activation Sheet

Like the journal, I have created this blank *Mind Over Muscle* Activation Sheet for you to photo copy and use on a daily basis. As you'll recall, the purpose of the sheet is to tap into the power of your emotions. I have even given you a space to outline your emotions about each goal, right there in black and white, so you don't forget. You have to decide what emotion you want to feel—self-confident, grateful, joyful, purposeful, worthy, energetic, etc.—and to feel this emotion in the present moment.

Remember, it's not a goals sheet or action plan; it's an Activation Sheet. We're doing just that; we're "activating" your emotional investment in each and every workout. Now go feel!

Date:
Time:

Overall Assessment of this Day: _____
_____
_____
_____
_____
_____
_____
_____
_____
_____

Assessment of the Day's Workout: _____
_____
_____
_____
_____
_____
_____
_____
_____
_____
_____
_____

Tomorrow's Goals: _____
_____
_____
_____
_____
_____
_____
_____
_____
_____
_____

Goal # 1: _____

Details of Goal # 1 (When, Why, How): _____
_____
_____

Emotion You Connect with Goal # 1: _____
_____
_____
_____

Goal # 2: _____

Details of Goal # 2 (When, Why, How): _____
_____
_____

Emotion You Connect with Goal # 2: _____
_____
_____
_____

Goal # 3: _____

Details of Goal # 1 (When, Why, How): _____
_____
_____

Emotion You Connect with Goal # 1: _____
_____
_____

APPENDIX C:
List of Foods to Choose

Early on in this book I said that I wanted you to have everything you needed—right here within these pages—to start, learn, and continue on the *Mind Over Muscle* Program. To that end I'm including here the food lists from which you can choose foods for your nutritional plan, outlined in Chapter 3.

While these lists are not complete, depending on the seasonal varieties of fruits and vegetables where you live and what's freshest in your neck of the woods, they are quite extensive and offer you a wide range of variety from which to choose:

Starchy Carbohydrates
(Eat with all five–six meals throughout the day)

Around 25-27 grams of carbohydrates per serving.
Men: Two servings per meal.
Women: One serving per meal.

FOOD ITEM	SERVING SIZE (measure dry)	GLYCEMIC INDEX	DESIRABLE
Old Fashioned Oats	½ cup dry	Low	Highly
Cream of Rice *	¼ cup dry	High	Good after workout only
Cream of Wheat	4 tablespoons dry	Medium	Good
Baked Potatoes	8 ounce cooked	Medium	Good
Sweet Potatoes	8 ounce cooked	Medium	Good
Rice (Brown Whole Grain)	½ cup cooked	Medium	Good
White Rice *	½ cup cooked	Medium	Good
Spaghetti	4 oz cooked	Low	Good in GI but too many carbs for a small serving.
Whole wheat flour bread	2 slices	High	Not a great choice but ok in moderation.
Corn	¾ cup	Medium	Good
Peas	1 cup	Medium	Good

Low GI=1-55 Medium GI=56-69 High GI=70-100

Simple Carbohydrates
(Eat one serving with Breakfast and one after workout as even though they are low to medium in GI, too many simple sugars in the diet throughout the day prevent fat loss)

Around 10 grams of carbohydrates per serving.

Men: Two servings per meal.

Women: One serving per meal.

FOOD ITEM	SERVING SIZE	GLYCEMIC INDEX	DESIRABLE
Apples	$^1/_2$	Low	Good
Oranges	$^1/_2$	Low	Good
Grapefruit	$^1/_2$	Low	Good
Cherries	7	Low	Good
Pears	$^1/_3$	Low	Good
Banana *	$^1/_3$	Medium	After Workout Only
Lemons	1	Low	Good
Cantaloupe	$^1/_4$ melon	High	After Workout Only
Strawberries	1 cup	1 cup	Good
Apricots	3	Medium	After Workout Only
Grapes	$^1/_2$ cup	Low	Good
Mango	$^1/_3$ cup	Medium	After Workout Only
Papaya	$^1/_2$ cup	Medium	After Workout Only

Low GI=1-55 Medium GI=56-69 High GI=70-100

Fibrous Carbohydrates

(Eat at least one serving with lunch and one serving with
dinner, though more can be consumed if desired)

Around 10 grams of carbohydrates per serving.

Men: Two servings per meal.

Women: One serving per meal.

FOOD ITEM	SERVING SIZE (measure cooked)	GLYCEMIC INDEX	DESIRABLE
Broccoli	1 cup	Low	Good
Green Beans	1 cup	Low	Good
Asparagus	12 spears or 1 cup	Low	Good
Lettuce	1 head raw	Low	Good
Tomatoes	2 raw	Low	Good

FOOD ITEM	SERVING SIZE (measure cooked)	GLYCEMIC INDEX	DESIRABLE
Green Peppers (chopped)	1-$\frac{1}{2}$ cup raw	Low	Good
Onions	$\frac{1}{2}$ cup	Low	Good
Mushrooms	1 cup	Low	Good
Cucumber sliced	3 cups	Low	Good
Cauliflower	2 cups	Low	Good
Spinach	4 cups	Low	Good
Cabbage	2 cups	Low	Good
Carrots	$\frac{1}{2}$ cup sliced	High	After Workout

Low GI=1-55 Medium GI=56-69 High GI=70-100

Proteins
(Eat with all five to six meals throughout the day)

Around 20-23 grams of protein per serving.

Men: 2 servings per meal.

Women: 1 serving per meal.

FOOD ITEM	SERVING SIZE (measure cooked)	GLYCEMIC INDEX	DESIRABLE
Chicken breast (skinless)	3 ounces	Low	Good
Turkey	3 ounces	Low	Good
Veal	3 ounces	Low	Good
Top Sirloin	3 ounces	Low	Good
Tuna	3 ounces	Low	Good
Wild Alaskan Salmon **	3 ounces	Low	Good
Egg Whites (in carton)	3 ounces	Low	Good
Whey Protein	3 ounces	Low	Good
Orange Roughy	3 ounces	Low	Good

All proteins are low in glycemic index and by combining a carbohydrate with a protein the combined glycemic index of the whole meal goes down as a result. The proteins included here were selected due to their low fat content and their digestibility.

NOTES: Avoid deli meats as they are high in sodium and if eating salmon, eliminate two servings of good fats.

Good Fats

Around 5 grams of fats per serving.

Men: One serving per meal.

Women: One serving in breakfast, lunch and dinner.

FOOD ITEM	SERVING SIZE	GLYCEMIC INDEX	DESIRABLE
Fish Oils	1 teaspoon	Low	Good
Flax Oils ***	1 teaspoon	Low	Good
Extra Virgin Olive Oil	1 teaspoon	Low	Good
Natural Peanut Butter	2 teaspoons	Low	Good

All fats are low in glycemic index and by combining a carbohydrate with a protein the combined glycemic index of the whole meal goes down as a result. The fats included here were selected due to their high essential fatty acids content and their health properties.

NOTES: Avoid cooking with flax oil as the heat degrades the oil. Bake and broil instead of frying. Also, if eating salmon, eliminate two servings of good fats as salmon is high in EFAs.

Resources

www.digitalmeditation.com

Featuring the exclusive AV3X technology; a multidimensional blending of mood-altering music, mesmerizing video effects, natural sounds, and pulsating light that actually tame the chaotic brainwaves caused by stress, anxiety, sleeplessness, and other intrusions. It's like nothing you've ever experienced!

www.fitnessbusinesscoach.com

A site for all health & fitness professionals looking to achieve their highest level of success & wealth—The Fitness Business Coaches will now help you sculpt your business wealthy.

www.getfitnow.com

A great source for all of your fitness equipment needs and home of the getfitnow.com discussion boards, where you can get support while on your quest for physical perfection.

www.losefatandgainmuscle.com

If you're looking for a companion resource that will truly help you lose fat & gain muscle, this is the website that people visit to finally achieve it!

www.mycustomworkout.com

The My Custom Workout programs make up the only fitness system designed to include absolutely everyone. This program was created to abolish the "one size fits all" approach to fitness. We have consciously included every individual while taking into consideration people's widely varied backgrounds and lifestyles. My Custom Workout programs customize individual, unique workouts for each specific lifestyle, filling a significant void in the fitness industry. Even more effective than one-on-one training, these customized modules allow innumerable individuals to achieve health and fitness, improving their well-being and self-image and giving them the dream body they've always desired.

www.trivelltechnique.com

A guide to yoga, relaxation, and other mind/body techniques from Lisa Trivell.

Works Cited

Introduction

"Belief in Exercise May Make It More Effective." Reuters. Accessed 11 March 2007
  <http://www.reuters.com/article/healthNews/idUSCOL37353320070213 >.

Chapter 1

Anthony, William P., E. Nick Maddox, and Walter Wheatley. *Envisionary Management: A Guide for Human Resource Professionals in Management Training and Development.* New York: Quorum Books, 1988.

Armstrong, D. M. *The Mind-Body Problem: An Opinionated Introduction.* Boulder, CO: Westview Press, 1999.

Benson, Herbert. "Mind-Body Pioneer." *Psychology Today,* May 2001: 56.

Csikszentmihaly, Mihaly. *Creativity: Flow and the Psychology of Discovery and Invention.* New York, NY: HarperCollins, 1997.

Gandee, Robert N., Helen Knierim, and Doris Mclittle-Marino. "Stress and Older Adults: A Mind-Body Relationship." *The Journal of Physical Education, Recreation & Dance* 69.9 (1998): 19+.

Goleman, Daniel, and Joel Gurin. *Mind Body Medicine: How to Use Your Mind for Better Health.* Consumer Reports Books, 1995.

Kason, Yvonne. *Farther Shores: Exploring How Near-Death, Kundalini and Mystical Experiences Can Transform Ordinary Lives,* Revised edition. Toronto: HarperCollins Publishers, 2000.

Leviton, Charles D., and Patti Leviton. "What Is Guided Imagery? The Cutting-Edge Process in Mind/body Medical Procedures." *Annals of the American Psychotherapy Association* 7.2 (2004): 22+.

Magnusson, Davis S., and Norman S. Endler, ed. *Personality at the Crossroads: Current Issues in Interactional Psychology.* Hillsdale, NJ: Lawrence Erlbaum Associates, 1977.

Mclean, Peter D., and Sheila R. Woody. *Anxiety Disorders in Adults: An Evidence-Based Approach to Psychological Treatment.* New York: Oxford University Press, 2001.

Okonski, Verna O. "Exercise as a Counseling Intervention." *Journal of Mental Health Counseling* 25.1 (2003): 45+.

Ornstein, Robert, and David Sobel. "The Healing Brain; Individuals with a Strong Sense of Belonging May Have Minds That Are Better Adapted to Preventing Disease." *Psychology Today* Mar. 1987: 48+.

Thayer, Robert E. *Calm Energy: How People Regulate Mood with Food and Exercise.* New York: Oxford University Press, 2003.

Chapter 2

Kiresuk, Thomas J., Aaron Smith, and Joseph E. Cardillo, eds., *Goal Attainment Scaling: Applications, Theory, and Measurement.* Hillsdale, NJ: Lawrence Erlbaum Associates, 1994: 3.

World Disease Weekly. November 2004.

Chapter 3

Thayer, Robert E. *Calm Energy: How People Regulate Mood with Food and Exercise.* New York: Oxford University Press, 2003: 65.

"Body Talk: Feeling Grumpy? Have a Banana! To Change Your Mood, Just Change Your Eating Habits—Tuck Into Foods That Will Make Your Life Easier." *The Mirror* (London, England) 28 Apr. 2005: 38

"Body Talk: Happy Meals; Feeling Down? Then Take a Good Look at Your Diet. The Latest Research Shows Eating Foods High in Omega-3 Can Put a Smile Back on Your Face." *The Mirror* (London, England)

"Body Talk: Ultimate Family Food Guide. Is Food Affecting Their Mood? Does Your Child Get a Portion Of Hyperactivity With Their Pizza? Here Are the Bad-Mood Foods to Leave Off the Menu." *The Mirror* (London, England) 21 Apr. 2005: 44.

Chapter 5

"The Importance of a Good Stretch." *Ebony* June 2002: 114.

About the Author

As a child, James Villepigue was anything but healthy and fit. Throughout high school, he was constantly getting bullied and wanted to leave school permanently. Luckily he had a great family, who helped him stay strong and influenced him to stay and stick it out. Now he's proud to hold certifications from the American Council On Exercise (ACE) as a certified personal trainer, the International Sports Sciences Association (ISSA) as a personal fitness trainer/counselor, the National Board Of Fitness Examiners (NBFE) as a TK, the Aerobics and Fitness Association of America (AFAA) as a personal fitness trainer/counselor and weight room certified trainer, the New York College of Oriental Medicine as a massage therapist, and the renowned Institute for Professional Empowerment Coaching (IPEC) as a life coach. He was also a strength and conditioning coach for the United States Karate Team.

Throughout his career, James has passionately kept up to date with the latest trends and rapid changes within the bodybuilding and fitness world. The adversity that once accompanied James Villepigue's life is not unlike the lives of so many people today. This led him to dedicate his life to helping others combat adversity and now make their fitness dreams and goals come true. In addition to writing the bestselling Body Sculpting Bible series of weight-training books for Hatherleigh Press, he provides empowerment/life coaching services to thousands of clients.

With *On-Line Fitness Training,* he works directly with you to create your ideal physique through telephone and e-mail correspondence. In the first stage, he assesses your current health and fitness condition. In the second stage, he pinpoints your goals and expectations. In the third stage, he creates a customized exercise routine for you and will follow-up regularly to keep you on track and keep the results coming along. With the *Empowerment/Life Coaching* service, he applies similar techniques to help you improve many different conditions in your life. You may also wish to combine the two services for a *Total Package.* The *Total Package* is a wonderful opportunity for you to make powerful, solid and life-long changes to every facet of your life.

Finally, James also offers a new program entitled "Fiscal Fitness Training: 5 Steps to Sculpting Your Business Wealthy" in which he draws on his own journey to the top of the fitness industry and translates that into a direct plan of action to help you take your business or career to the top of *your* industry. If you're ready to seriously experience happiness, success, and abundance, stop letting fear hold you back and get started right now.

If you are interested in working with James on a one-on-one basis, please visit www.lifecoachjames.com. When you visit the site, enter the code words "coach me" in the prompt box and you will receive a special complimentary session, only available to the readers of *Mind Over Muscle.*

Million Man (*By*) March

My Journey to Helping One Million People by March 2008

Hi, my name is James Villepigue. Many of you might already know of me or about my bestselling fitness series, The Body Sculpting Bibles. For those of you who are new to both me and my fitness books, over the last seven years, I have written over 18 books, creating one of the most successful fitness book series in history. I've helped literally hundreds of thousands of people, from all over the world and all walks of life, transform their bodies into masterpieces. My Body Sculpting Bible books have been proven to work wonders, as they have literally changed people's lives.

I am now dedicated to helping an additional one million people and I could really use your help to reach my goal. Please note: I am not asking you to help me without giving you something VERY valuable in return. Now, truth be told, many of my fellow fitness experts and online marketers are not going to be happy with what I'm going to offer, as they feel that giving valuable information for free makes it harder to sell that valuable information--but I see this as being a huge benefit to everyone. The more people who show interest in fitness and a desire to shape up, the more it benefits everyone, right?

I have just finished my latest book, entitled *Emotional Fitness: Real Problems, Real Solutions*. It is, without question, one of my favorite projects to date. Just as we need exercise to strengthen and help the body, we also need emotional exercise to strengthen the mind. Use them together and you now have an arsenal of tools to create total life balance and happiness.

My original plan was to publish the book and sell it for $19.95. But now I have decided to give you the book, for free, as a way of showing my gratitude for your support.

Please take a moment and visit www.mindovermusclebonus.com. There you'll see an opt-in contact box. Fill in your name and email address and hit "download." When you do, you will automatically be brought to an encrypted download page where you will right click and hit "Save Target As." This will allow you to download your free copy of *Zone Tone II*. I guarantee that when you utilize some of the tools, tactics, and techniques that I describe, you will absolutely be enthralled with the outcomes.

In addition, if you fill in the box with an additional five names and email addresses of people you know who also love fitness, you will be brought to a page where you will once again, right click and hit "Save Target As." There you will be able to download an additional bestselling book, entitled *Goal Mining: The Strike It Rich Formula for Achieving Virtually Anything!*

Well, that's it for now. I thank you from the bottom of my heart for your support and if you have absolutely any questions about your free gifts, feel free to email me at millionmanbymarch@gmail.com

All My Best,
James Villepigue

International Bestselling Author, Fitness Expert & Success Coach
www.jvfitness.com
www.fitnessbusinesscoach.com
www.lifecoachjames.com
www.thegoalbook.com
Believe & Achieve! Featured Fitness Trainer of "The Regis & Kelly Show"